153.—

NEONATAL SKIN

DERMATOLOGY

series editors

Charles D. Calnan

Consultant Dermatologist
University of London—British Postgraduate Medical Federation
St. John's Hospital for Diseases of the Skin
London, England

Howard Maibach

Department of Dermatology
University of California School of Medicine
Ambulatory Care Center 342
San Francisco, California

Volume 1 Neonatal Skin: Structure and Function, *edited by Howard Maibach and Edward K. Boisits*

Additional Volumes in Preparation

Volume 2 Allergic Contact Dermatitis to Simple Compounds, *edited by Gilles Dupuis and Claude Benezra*

NEONATAL SKIN

Structure and Function

edited by
HOWARD MAIBACH

Department of Dermatology
University of California School of Medicine
Ambulatory Care Center 342
San Francisco, California

EDWARD K. BOISITS

Department of Skin Biology
Johnson and Johnson Baby Products Company
Skillman, New Jersey

MARCEL DEKKER, INC.   New York and Basel

Library of Congress Cataloging in Publication Data
Main entry under title:

Neonatal skin.

   (Dermatology ; v. 1)
   Includes indexes.
   1. Pediatric dermatology. 2. Skin.
3. Infants (Newborn)–Physiology. I. Maibach,
Howard I. II. Boisits, Edward K., [date].
III. Series: Dermatology (Marcel Dekker, Inc.) ;
v. 1. [DNLM: 1. Skin–Anatomy and histology.
2. Skin-Physiology. 3. Skin diseases–In infancy
and childhood. 4. Infant, Newborn. W1 DE5084 v.1/
WR 102 N438]
RJ511.N4 1982   618.92'5   82-10081
ISBN 0-8247-1860-7

MARCEL DEKKER, INC.
270 Madison Avenue, New York, New York 10016

Current printing (last digit):
10 9 8 7 6 5 4 3 2 1

PRINTED IN THE UNITED STATES OF AMERICA

Series Introduction

Many dermatologists along with other doctors and scientists were surprised by the views of an eminent medical Nobel Prize winner who said that all the major discoveries in biology have been made and little can be expected from now on. The scientific achievements of the past 40 years, even in relation to medicine alone, have been so phenomenal that one may wonder if there is anything of importance left for future generations. The same attitude may be taken with regard to medical books, and especially in relation to dermatology. So much has been written over the past 30 years that one may question whether there are any books of value left to be written. Nothing could be further from the truth.

The functions of medical journals and medical books are different. As the number, diversity, and output of journals expands, so does the need for medical books; this is as true for dermatology as for any other branch of medicine. And it is equally true for the subdivisions of dermatology. Some doctors may regret increasing subspecialization within a single branch such as dermatology, but it is a reflection of the steady and inevitable increase in knowledge within the subject. Specialized clinics and departments are now the norm rather than the exception within many university dermatological centers. Their outward manifestation is the growth of subspecialty journals in relation to such subjects as dermatological surgery and oncology, contact dermatitis and occupational dermatoses, microbiology, and pediatric dermatology.

The subdivision of subjects such as dermatology today is a reflection of the subdivision of internal medicine 40 years ago, and it produces similar opposing groups of antagonists. The dearth of the general dermatologist may come to be mourned in the same way as has the dearth of the general physician. But the practical clinical dermatologist and the physician who has responsibility for the care of patients with skin disease will usually depend more on books than on journals when he/she needs help. This is particularly true of dermatologists who work away from university centers, especially outside Western Europe and North America, and who constitute a "silent majority." Although there is still a place for the comprehensive textbook, the growth of specialist books has shown the need for such condensation of recent specialist information.

The Medical Division of Marcel Dekker, Inc. has decided to meet this need with a selective series of books on particular branches of dermatology, especially in fields which have frontiers with more than one scientific discipline. The emphasis, however, will be on the information requirements of dermatologists whose responsibilities involve not only the clinical care of patients, but also extend to education and research.

Charles D. Calnan, M.D.
Howard Maibach, M.D.

Foreword

"Nothing is constant but change" applies in full force to the structures and functions of the human body. It is likely that such changes occur incessantly at all ages. During most of adult life the changes may be subtle, not readily discernible. There are, however, certain periods during which the changes in both structure and function are obvious, fundamental, decisive. Such periods of obvious changes occur during fetal life, during neonatal or perinatal life, during adolescence, and during senescence.

There have been relatively few publications about perinatal changes of the skin, that huge organ which is among those most affected by the monumental event of birth and the demands of the immediate postnatal period. Prenatally, the human skin has been immersed in a virtually sterile fluid maintained at constant temperature and pressure, has been shrouded in darkness, buffered against shocks, and protected against friction. At birth, all this changes. The skin is quite suddenly exposed to dry air, light, to substantial swings in environmental temperature, shocks and friction, a hail of microorganisms, innumerable natural and synthetic chemicals, washing and drying, clothing, and to countless other new outrageous onslaughts.

If the human skin had not to a considerable extent prepared itself *in utero* to meet these strange new environmental exposures, none of us would survive for more than a very brief time. But *in utero* the skin has formed a watertight horny layer without which the newborn infant would soon dry up and shrivel away. And *in utero* the fetus's sebaceous glands have formed and functioned, some of its corneocytes have combined to make another protective mantle, a covering that is lubricating, insulating, and probably antimicrobial.

The newborn infant, as it becomes an endothermic being, needs to conserve heat. Cooling by means of eccrine sweat is therefore not an immediate necessity. In contrast to the intrauterine activity of the sebaceous glands, the eccrine apparatus, though fully formed and patent, does not secrete and deliver sweat until two to eighteen days after birth. Therefore, beginning in fetal life and continuing during infancy, the protective structures and mechanisms develop seriatim. All those that become available and functional later are by no means fully formed and fully competent in the neonatal skin.

In 1935, Lewis Webb Hill and I, pointing out the differences between the infantile, childhood, and young adult phases of atopic dermatitis wrote:

> The infant is not merely a small man;
> he is a different sort of small man.*

In *Neonatal Skin: Structure and Function,* editors Howard Maibach and Edward K. Boisits, together with 16 other distinguished investigators present their findings showing how and when the various neonatal skin structures and functions develop and at what rate each progresses toward its more mature state. The delayed development of certain physical, biochemical, immunological, and other properties makes the neonatal and infant skin react differently from that of the older individual. This brings about a distinctive dermatology of infancy. There are skin diseases essentially confined or peculiar to infants and young children: diaper rash, granuloma glutaeale infantum, scalded skin syndrome, Leiner's erythroderma desquamativa, and Ritter von Rittershain's dermatitis exfoliativa, to name a few. In addition, many skin diseases common to both infant and adult can, in the newborn, take on a characteristically different appearance, have a different prognosis and course, demand different approaches to diagnosis, prevention, and management, and differ in still other respects from the same dermatoses in older patients.

It follows that *Neonatal Skin: Structure and Function* will be invaluable to all who deal with the health of neonates and infants. Between the covers of this book there is a wealth of information not assembled elsewhere—information useful to embryologists, pediatricians, obstetricians, dermatologists, family physicians, and many others.

Marion B. Sulzberger, M.D.
Emeritus Professor
University of California Medical School
San Francisco, California

---

*Evolution of atopic dermatitis. Arch. Dermatol. Syphilol. 32:451-463, 1935.

Preface

Neonatal human skin is taken very much for granted. It is so soft, so smooth, and so perfect! Unfortunately, until recently, there has been little systematic study of its structure and function. This volume summarizes previous experience as well as considerable new information.

The book starts with a complete description of the histology and ultrastructure of neonatal skin. Next, Drs. Green and Pochi delineate the structure and function of neonatal skin appendages: the eccrine and sebaceous glands. Noninvasive techniques utilized to determine aspects of skin function in the neonate are discussed in Chapters 4-9. The techniques include determination of transepidermal water loss, carbon dioxide emission rates, and oxygen diffusion. These chapters define not only the relevant physiology, but current information on the advantages and limitations of today's technology.

The next two chapters review knowledge of the quantitative aspects of percutaneous penetration in relation to current data in adults. Neonatal cutaneous microbiology with regard to normal and diseased skin is then summarized by Drs. Leyden, Aly, and associates.

The cutaneous dermatotoxicology section includes diaper dermatitis, allergic contact dermatitis in children, and the complex factors involved in diaper and plastic occlusion. In the final chapter, a concise overview of neonatal cutaneous disorders is provided.

Hopefully, this summary will stimulate further investigation. There is much to learn.

Howard Maibach, M.D.
Edward K. Boisits, Ph.D.

Contributors

Raza Aly, Ph.D. Associate Professor of Dermatology and Microbiology, Department of Dermatology, University of California Medical School, San Francisco, California

Ted L. Blaney, Master's in Chemical Engineering Staff Engineer, The Procter and Gamble Company, Cincinnati, Ohio

Edward K. Boisits, Ph.D., M.S. Assistant Manager, Skin Biology, Johnson and Johnson Baby Products Company, Skillman, New Jersey

Ernst Epstein, M.D. Clinical Associate Professor, Department of Dermatology, University of California Medical Center, San Francisco, California

L. B. Fisher, Ph.D. Johnson and Johnson Baby Products Company, Skillman, New Jersey

Marvin Green, M.D. Professor, Department of Pediatrics, School of Medicine, State University of New York, Stony Brook, New York

Karen A. Holbrook, Ph.D. Associate Professor and Vice Chairman, Biological Structure; Adjunct Associate Professor of Medicine (Dermatology), University of Washington School of Medicine, Seattle, Washington

Sidney Hurwitz, M.D. Associate Clinical Professor, Pediatrics and Dermatology, Yale University School of Medicine, New Haven, Connecticut

William E. Jordan, Ph.D. Research Chemist, Research and Development, The Procter and Gamble Company, Miami Valley Laboratories, Cincinnati, Ohio

James J. Leyden, M.D. Associate Professor of Dermatology, Department of Dermatology, University of Pennsylvania, Philadelphia, Pennsylvania

John J. McCormack, B.S. Scientist, Basic Research, Johnson and Johnson Baby Products Company, Skillman, New Jersey

Howard Maibach, M.D. Professor, Department of Dermatology, University of California Medical School, San Francisco, California

Peter E. Pochi, M.D. Professor, Department of Dermatology and Evans Memorial Department of Clinical Research, University Hospital, Boston University Medical Center, Boston, Massachusetts

John W. Severinghaus, M.D., F.F.A.R.C.S. Professor, Department of Anesthesia, University of California Medical School, San Francisco, California

Henry R. Shinefield, M.D. Chief of Pediatrics, Clinical Professor of Pediatrics and Dermatology, San Francisco Kaiser Permanente Medical Center, University of California Medical School, San Francisco, California

Hans T. Versmold, M.D. Professor, Head of the Division of Neonatology, University of Munich, Munich, Federal Republic of Germany

Ronald C. Wester, Ph.D. Research Dermatologist, Department of Dermatology University of California Medical School, San Francisco, California

Donald R. Wilson, M.A. Staff Research Associate, Department of Dermatology, University of California Medical School, San Francisco, California

Contents

NEONATAL SKIN

STRUCTURE

1

A Histological Comparison of Infant and Adult Skin

KAREN A. HOLBROOK
University of Washington School of Medicine, Seattle, Washington

The neonatal period of life is a distinctive phase in the biology of skin, characterized by unique functional properties and associated clinical peculiarities (often transient), but which appears to have few remarkable structural features specific only to this stage of skin development.

Percutaneous absorption is elevated in newborn skin [1] and transepidermal water loss is diminished [2], yet the thickness and integrity of the stratum corneum are equivalent to adult. The sweating response is delayed at birth [1] even though the sweat glands are structurally mature and the ducts are patent. That many of these functional properties must be explained primarily on a physiological basis, and not by structural qualities, is also reflected by the absence of a specific literature on the structure of newborn skin. With the exception of a few textbook chapters [3-5] and survey papers [1] devoted to neonatal skin biology in general, there have been no morphological studies undertaken specifically to compare the structure of the epidermis, dermis, and epidermal appendages in newborn and adult skin. The present study was designed to meet this need. In order to understand the position of neonatal skin morphology in the total sequence of cutaneous development, neonatal and adult skin were also compared histologically and ultrastructurally with skin from premature infants.

MATERIALS AND METHODS

Skin was obtained, within the first few hours or days after birth, with an electric biopsy drill from the arm of three full-term, newborns and from several body regions (arm, leg, back, abdomen, cheek, forehead, scalp, nipple, axilla, finger) of a fourth, term infant. Samples were also taken from the edge of a mid-line incision in the trunk of each of two premature infants born at 30 and 32 weeks of age. Site-matched material was biopsied from several adults in the age range of 20-35 years. All samples were fixed in Karnovsky's fixative [6] for 2 hr at room temperature, washed in buffer, and postfixed for an additional hour in 1% OsO_4 in distilled water. For light and transmission electron microscopy, portions of the biopsy were dehydrated through a graded series of alcohols and embedded in Epon [7]. Thin sections were stained with 1% phosphotungstic acid (PTA), uranyl acetate, and lead citrate and viewed in a Philips 201 transmission electron microscope. Whole mount preparations for scanning electron microscopy were dehydrated through the alcohol series into a second series of alcohol-Genesolv (Freon 113) in increasing concentrations of freon to 100% Genesolv. These specimens were dried in a critical point dryer with Freon 13 as the transitional fluid [8], mounted on aluminum stubs, sputter-coated with gold palladium alloy, and viewed in an Etec Autoscan SEM operated at 20 kV in the secondary electron mode.

RESULTS AND DISCUSSION

Regional Variation

It is difficult to compare similar structures in skin from the adult, term newborn, and premature infant by using a few site-selected specimens, because nearly every structure in the skin expresses some degree of regional specificity. Figure 1 illustrates the extent to which this structural variation can exist from one part of the body to another in an individual of a given age. However, for specific comparisons of structure in the epidermis, dermis, and epidermal appendages among the three age groups, it was necessary to limit the samples to a few regions. For this purpose we have chosen skin from the arm of the term newborn and adult and from the abdomen of the premature infant. Abdominal skin was used from the last individuals because of limited availability of tissue but this tissue was believed to have similar enough characteristics with the skin of the arm to permit reasonable comparisons to be made (compare Fig 1d, g).

Full Thickness Skin

Thickness of the skin, as determined by measurements with a caliper micrometer, is dependent upon the bulk of dermal connective tissue and the accumulation of subcutaneous fat. At any stage of skin development, this measurement varies with the region of the body (Fig. 1). In the infant, thickness is also related to the birthweight and, specifically in the neonatal period, can vary at a given site

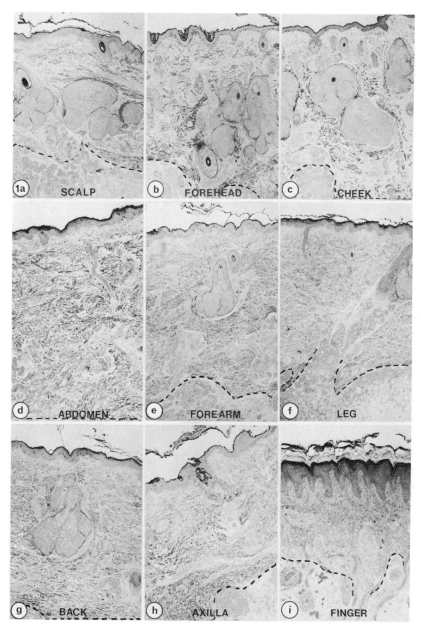

Figure 1 Full-thickness skin samples obtained from multiple body regions of a term newborn infant. Note differences in the thickness of the epidermis and dermis, density of sebaceous glands, and configuration of the dermal epidermal junction (X 75).

5

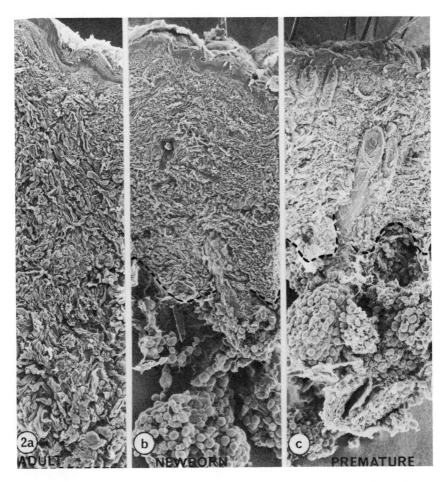

Figure 2 Scanning electron micrographs of full-thickness skin showing a thicker and coarser dermis in the adult tissue and a clear separation between the papillary and reticular dermis. The lines emphasize the junction between the dermis and hypodermis (× 100).

depending upon the sex [9]. Figure 2 shows a comparison of the full-thickness skin from the arm of an adult (a) and a full-term neonate (b), and the abdomen of a premature infant (c). Lines have been drawn to demarcate the dermis from hypodermis so that the average measurements of 2.1 mm (a), 1.2 mm (b), and 0.9 mm (c), respectively, express a lower value than would be measured with a

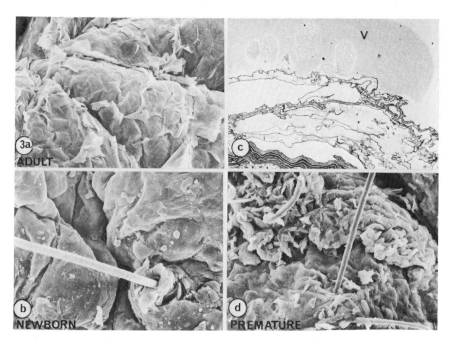

Figure 3 Scanning electron micrographs of the epidermal surface. The skin surface of the adult (a) appears drier than the vernix-coated surface of either newborn (b and d); adult squames are larger (X 350). Transmission electron micrograph through the epidermal surface of the term newborn (c). The surface material (vernix –V) looks like sebum and cellular debris (compare with Fig. 17) (X 4100).

caliper, and which, clearly, are dependent upon the amount of dermal connective tissue.

Epidermis

The dry, scaly surface of the adult skin may be compared in the scanning electron micrographs of Figure 3 with the greasy, vernix-coated skin of the full-term newborn and premature infant. The presence of vernix caseosa on the epidermal surface of the premature and term newborn reflects activity of the sebaceous glands in late prenatal stages and, for a limited period, after birth. These glands develop in the second trimester [10,11] and secrete sebum which accumulates on the body surface along with shed lanugo hairs, desquamated and decomposed periderm and epidermal cells. This material persists on the general body surface during the first several days of neonatal life and explains, in part, the many similarities between surface lipids in the newborn and the adult [12-14]. The submicroscopic structure of the vernix is similar to the structure of the lipid contained within maturing cells of the sebaceous gland (compare Figs. 3c and 17); other particulate material within the vernix is suggestive of decomposed cellular debris (Fig. 3c).

An even more vivid impression of the relative dryness of the adult skin when compared with the hydrated skin of the term newborn and premature baby is obtained from the scanning electron micrographs of sections through the epidermis (Fig. 4a-c). Individual layers of adult stratum corneum appeared to separate from one another (Fig. 4a), but in the term newborn, the stratum corneum separated primarily as a unit or as adherent sheets of multiple corneal layers (Fig. 4b). In the premature baby, only single cells or clusters of stratum corneum cells appeared loose at the epidermal surface (Fig. 4c); the majority of the stratum corneum, instead, was not loosened by the various reagents used in fixation and dehydration. This image gives a visual impression of the "gelatinous" quality which has been used to describe the texture of the premature skin (Fig. 4c).

The thickness of the epidermis, numbers and shapes of the cell layers, density of keratin filaments, frequency of desmosomes along cell borders, and extent of pigmentation were compared among samples of premature, term newborn, and adult skin. Figures 4-6 show a comparison of total epidermal thickness in light, scanning, and transmission electron micrographs. The thickness of the epidermis (50 μm ± SD) as well as the number of cells in each epidermal compartment (stratum corneum, stratum granulosum, etc.) were equivalent in the adult and term newborn (Figs. 5a,b and 6a,b). Except for the smaller and more uniform size of the horny cell in the newborn [15], the structural properties of these cells, the number of cell layers (15.2 ± 2.8 SD), and the thickness (9.3 μm ± 2.6 SD) of the stratum corneum were identical when compared with the adult. We could not substantiate, therefore, the suggestion that the newborn stratum corneum is thicker than adult, presumably as a consequence of impaired desquamation of the epidermis in utero. Granular and spinous cell layers in adult and full-term newborn epidermis also were equivalent in cell shape, density, and organization of the keratin filaments, and abundance of desmosomal junctions (Fig. 7a,b). Keratinocytes in the basal epidermal layer of the newborns showed fewer melanosome complexes than were seen in any of the adult specimens (Fig. 8a,b). Melanin production is low in the newborn [1] even though the mean number of melanocytes per square millimeter of epidermis is similar to that of an older child or an adult [16,17].

Several features were contrasted, however, between this structure of the premature and term newborn/adult epidermis. First, the entire epidermis was

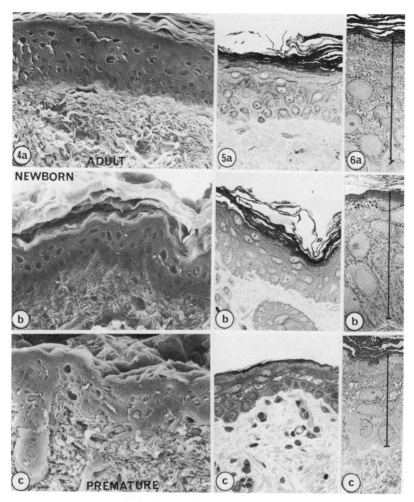

Figure 4 Scanning electron micrographs through the epidermis. Compare the separation of stratum corneum layers among the three specimens. The epidermis of the premature is thinner than either of the other specimens and appears more "gelatinous." Intradermal and intraepidermal portions of the sweat duct are seen in (c). Note the relative flat dermal-epidermal junction in all specimens (X 600).

Figures 5 and 6 Photomicrographs (Fig. 5) and electron micrographs (Fig. 6) showing the comparative thickness of epidermis in all three age groups (5a-c, X 550; 6a-c, X 1800).

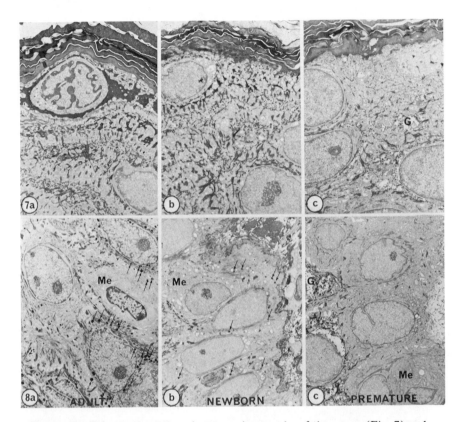

Figures 7 and 8 Transmission electron micrographs of the upper (Fig. 7) and lower (Fig. 8) layers of the epidermis. Adult and term newborn granular and spinous cells are equivalent in numbers of desmosomes and density of keratin filaments (Fig. 7a,b). Fewer and smaller filament bundles are apparent in the cytoplasm of the premature infant granular and spinous cells (c). Remnants of glycogen (G) persist in the cytoplasm of these cell layers. Basal keratinocytes of the adult contain many melanosome complexes (arrows) by comparison with the few observed in term newborn basal keratinocytes; an absence of melanosome complexes is apparent in cells from the premature infant. Melanosomes (Me) are seen in all samples (7a-c, × 5000; 8a-c, × 3750).

thinner (27.4 μm ± 6.4 SD) (Figs. 4c, 5c, and 6c) and cells of all strata were more compressed. The stratum corneum consisted of only a few cell layers (5.6 μm ± 0.8 SD) and as a consequence was markedly thinner (4.1 μm ± 1.0 SD) than that of older specimens. These observations may correlate with the clinical findings of a marked increase in skin permeability of premature (28- to 37-week-old) neonates to drugs applied topically within the first few days after birth [18]. Smaller bundles of keratin filaments and fewer desmosomes were evident among the granular and spinous cells (Fig. 7c). Large accumulations of glycogen, a distinctly fetal characteristic, still persisted in the cytoplasm of the spinous layer cells, but this material was poorly preserved by tissue processing, leaving apparently empty spaces where extracted. Melanocytes were recognized among basal cells but did not contain mature melanosomes (Fig. 8c) and melanosome complexes were not visible in the cytoplasm of keratinocytes. At this age the numbers of melanosomes per square millimeter is about one-third of those present at birth but, in contrast with our observations, they have been found by others to contain mature melanin granules [16].

Dermal-Epidermal Junction

In most regions of the body of the term newborn the junction between the dermis and epidermis was flat (Fig. 1), however, the entire hemidesmosome-basal lamina structural complex (Fig. 9a) was formed as completely in this tissue as in the adult (compare Fig. 9b,c). There were no apparent differences either in the quantity of basal cell keratin filaments associated with the hemidesmosomes, anchoring filaments/fibrils that bind the epidermis to the basal lamina/dermal collagen, density of collagen fibrils in the papillary dermis immediately subjacent to the epidermis, or in the frequency of hemidesmosomes per equivalent linear distance. On the basis of junction morphology, therefore, it is not clear why there is a greater tendency for blistering in the normal newborn [1]. When structural anomalies are present, however, in the junction above [19] or below [20] the basal lamina, or in the numbers of hemidesmosomes per linear measurement, as in newborn infants with epidermolytic bullous disorders, blistering is a correlated phenomenon.

In the premature infant one might anticipate a tendency to blister, assuming epidermal-dermal instability can be predicted from morphology of the junction. Although all of the structural components of the hemidesmosome were formed at this stage, the junctions were smaller and spaced less frequently along the basal cell border (Fig. 9d). The papillary dermis beneath the basal lamina was more edematous and had a looser organization of fine collagen fibers, hence would be presumed to provide a less secure anchoring site than the papillary dermis of either the term newborn or adult.

Aside from the surface coating of vernix and limited pigmentation, the epidermis of the newborn had no remarkable differences in structure from that of the adult when identical sites were compared. By contrast the epidermis of the young premature baby (30-32 weeks) had characteristics more similar to newly keratinized, fetal epidermis: thin total thickness, fewer and thinner layers of

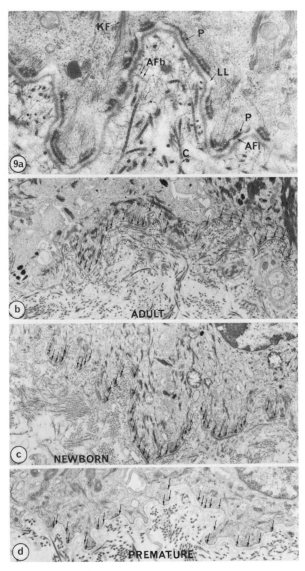

Figure 9 Junctions at the dermal-epidermal border. The structural details of the hemidesmosome are shown in (a): keratin filaments (KF), attachment plaque (P), lamina lucida (LL), anchoring filaments (AFi), basal lamina (BL), anchoring fibrils (AFb), papillary dermal collagen (C). Arrows indicate the frequency of hemidesmosomes at this boundary (a, × 34,500; b, × 10,800; c, × 9100; d, × 15,400).

stratum corneum, cytoplasmic glycogen, fewer desmosomes and hemidesmosomes, and less well developed keratin filament bundles.

Dermis

In the adult there was a clear demarcation between the papillary and reticular dermis on the basis of size of collagen fiber bundles (Figs. 2a, 10a, 12a). By the same criterion, there was a subdivision within the papillary dermis into a finely organized, subepidermal, collagen meshwork and, adjacent to the reticular dermis, a zone of more coarse fiber bundles (Figs. 10a and 12a). Large-diameter fiber bundles of the reticular dermis progressively increased in size toward the hypodermis (Figs. 2a, 11a,a', 13a). A fine fibrous net was also evident beneath the epidermis in the term newborn and premature skin, but the boundary between papillary and reticular dermis in these two age groups was less defined because of a more gradual transition in fiber bundle size and a final fiber bundle size that was considerably smaller than that of the adult (Figs. 10b,c, 12b,c). From the series of scanning electron micrographs in Figures 10 and 11, it is clear that fewer differences exist among the age groups in the organization of the papillary dermis than in the reticular dermis. Collagen bundles in the reticular dermis of the premature infant skin were only slightly larger than in the papillary dermis and were markedly smaller than reticular bundles from either of the other age groups (Figs. 10c, 11c, 12c, 13c). Fiber bundles in the reticular dermis of the full-term neonate were intermediate in size, larger than those in the premature infant, but smaller than any of the fiber bundles in either the uppermost or deepest regions of the adult (Figs. 11b and 13b). Note the extensive amount of regional variation that can exist in the thickness of the dermis, and the density and size of collagen bundles (Fig. 1).

At the light microscopic level, marked differences were seen among the age groups in the quantity and size of elastic fibers in the dermis. In the adult, the majority of the elastic connective tissue was distributed within the reticular dermis where large coarse fibers intertwined with collagen fiber bundles (Fig. 13a). Smaller bundles were present in the papillary dermis (Fig. 12a), although they were more obvious when this region was studied with the transmission electron microscope (Fig. 14a). It has been demonstrated that the elastic fibers in the papillary region are present in more variable states of maturity [21] (dependent on the ratio of the microfibrillar and amorphous, electron-dense elastin components), while those of the reticular dermis are fully formed and have a dense elastin matrix in which microfibrils are embedded almost imperceptibly (Fig. 15a). Elastic fibers were distributed in the reticular dermis of the term newborn in a pattern similar to the adult, but the fibers were considerably finer in diameter and less mature in structure (compare Figs. 13a,b, 14b, 15b). Elastic fibers were less apparent in the papillary dermis of these individuals at the light micro-

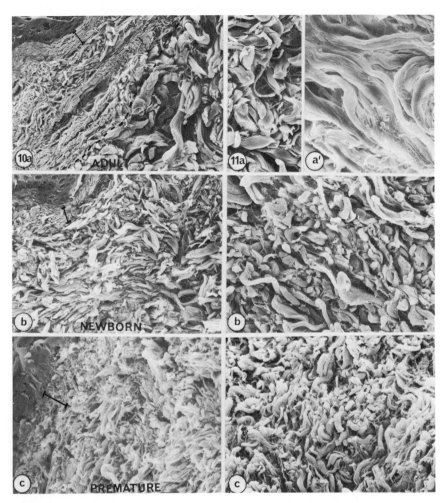

Figures 10 and 11 Scanning electron micrographs of the papillary dermis (PD) (Fig. 10) and reticular (RD) (Fig. 11) dermis. In the adult, the PD is subdivided into a fine subepidermal net (—) and a more coarse zone. The RD of the adult has intermediate-sized fiber bundles proximal to the PD (11a) but the bundles become increasingly larger toward the hypodermis (11a'). A subepidermal net is seen in the PD of the newborn but the distinction between PD and RD is unclear as the fiber bundles in the RD are smaller than either zone of the adult RD (11b). The RD from the premature infant is finely textured and more nearly comparable to the PD in the fiber bundle size (10c and 11c) (X 525).

14

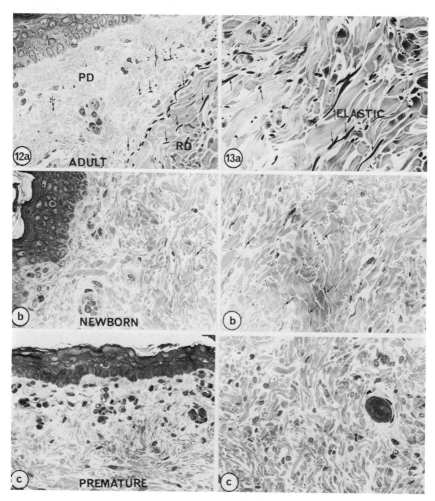

Figures 12 and 13 Light micrographs of the papillary dermis (PD) (Fig. 12) and reticular dermis (RD) (Fig. 13). In the adult only, note the distinct boundary between the PD and RD. Elastic fibers are large and dense in the adult (Fig. 13a, arrows), small and fine in the term newborn (13b), and indistinguishable in the premature infant (13c). The RD is markedly more cellular in the premature infant than either the term newborn or adult (× 450).

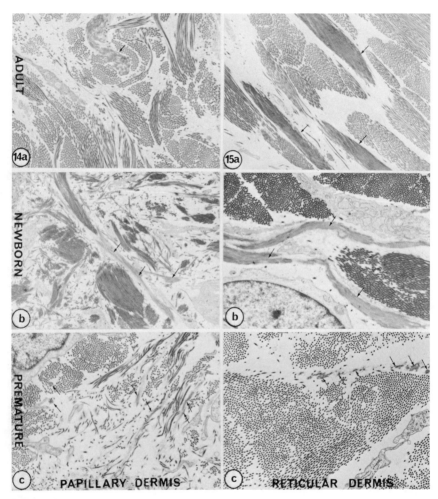

Figures 14 and 15 Elastic fibers (arrows) in the papillary (PD) dermis (Fig. 14) and reticular dermis (RD) (Fig. 15). Immature fibers are seen in the PD of skin from each age group, but the fibers vary in size and complexity. More elastin is associated with the microfibrils in the adult PD. Compare the large, dense elastic fibers in the adult RD (15a), the finer, less dense fibers in newborn RD (15b) and the fine wisps of microfibrils and sparse elastin in the premature RD (15c) (14a, × 9300; 14b, × 4400; 14c, × 9300; 15a, × 4400; 15b × 6500; 15c, × 9300).

16

scopic level but were easily recognized ultrastructurally as bundles of microfibrils with minimal amounts of elastin (Fig. 14b). The paucity of elastin accounts for their poor stainability and visualization histologically. Elastic fibers were not recognized in either zone of the dermis of the premature infants by light microscopy (Figs. 12c and 13c). By electron microscopy, however, very fine strands of immature elastic fibers were seen in both zones (Figs. 14c and 15c).

Elastic fibers are first secreted in the reticular dermis in the fetal skin around 22 weeks of estimated gestational age (EGA) (considerably later than the collagen fibrils) as short, granular fibers or as a network of finely branching fibers [22] that lack the elastin component. At approximately 28 weeks EGA, elastic fibers appear in the papillary dermis. Various accounts differ as to the maturity of elastin at birth; some studies have shown that the fibers have staining properties at birth which are indistinguishable from adult elastic fibers [22], while others, in concurrence with the present study, demonstrate that elastic fibers in the newborn have less amorphous elastin than the adult [23], and, in fact, may not become fully adultlike in structure until 3 years after birth.

A final comparison in dermal structure among the three age groups is in the numbers of cells within the connective tissue matrix. In adult skin, typically, the papillary dermis is more cellular (Fig. 12a) than the reticular dermis where few fibroblastic cells are present, localized primarily around blood vessels (Fig. 13a). By comparison, more fibroblastic cells were evident in the reticular dermis of the term newborn skin (Fig. 13b) which presumably is still actively synthesizing matrix proteins. Fibroblasts were most abundant in the reticular dermis of premature skin (Fig. 13c); in this tissue substantial bulk is yet to be accumulated in both collagen and elastic fiber populations.

In many respects, the organization, structure, and composition of the dermis in the term newborn has features intermediate between those of the adult and the premature infant. This is not surprising when one considers that the connective tissue components of the dermis have structural, kinetic, and biochemical age-related changes throughout life.

Epidermal Appendages

Hair Follicles and Sebaceous Glands: Hair follicles were not studied in any systematic manner as hair is fully formed in individuals of all age groups and varies markedly depending upon the individual, the region sampled, and the stage of the hair cycle of the particular follicle examined (Fig. 1). In the premature infant and in some full-term infants, fine lanugo hairs cover the body. These are soft, fine, poorly pigmented hairs that lack a medulla and have limited growth potential. An example of lanugo hair is seen in the full-thickness specimen from the trunk of a premature infant (Fig. 2c). Such follicles extend deeply into the subcutaneous fat, ensheathed by connective tissue

arranged in circular and longitudinal layers. Lanugo hairs are usually shed in the full-term infant and replaced by vellus hairs [1], which are replaced on the scalp by coarse, more densely pigmented terminal hairs. Growth of scalp hair before birth is usually synchronous, but modulated by sex, age, and nutritional status of the fetus [24]. Most of the follicles are in the anagen phase of activity, although this will vary according to the region of the scalp and the sex and hair color of the individual [25-27]. During the subsequent months a greater numbers of hairs become medullated and dyssynchrony of hair growth ensues [25, 26].

Sebaceous glands are active in utero (see p. 70) and during the end of the third trimester secrete disintegrated, lipid-filled cells in progressively greater numbers into the amniotic fluid. These cells stain orange or brown with Nile blue sulfate and, when counted and compared with the blue staining squames, serve as an index of fetal maturity [28]. At birth the sebaceous glands are large and well-developed over the entire skin surface. As in the adult, they exhibit significant differences in size and degree of lobulation depending upon the region of the body (Fig. 1). They continue to be active during the neonatal period under the influence of maternal androgens acquired transplacentally [12], then undergo involution and remain in a quiescent state, producing only small amounts of sebum, until puberty. Typical characteristics of the lipogenic cells in sebaceous glands were seen most clearly in the premature tissue, although the lipid was preserved to greater advantage in term newborn and adult skin (Figs. 16 and 17). In skin from all three age groups examined, sebaceous glands had a peripheral zone of mitotically active cells that showed no evidence of lipid synthesis and accumulation, an intermediate zone of cells in which the cytoplasm was dominated by smooth endoplasmic reticulum, lipid vesicles and lysosomal vacuoles (autophagosomes), and a central region of cells distended with coalesced lipid vesicles, to the degree that the remainder of the cytoplasm was nearly obliterated (Figs. 16 and 17).

Cells in the proximal portion of the sebaceous duct also can synthesize sebum (Fig. 18), but as the duct approaches the infundibulum of the follicle distally its cells become more completely keratinized.

Eccrine Sweat Glands: The eccrine sweat glands are formed and the ducts are patent by the end of the second trimester [29] although sweating does not occur in a premature infant until several days after birth [1]; even in a full-term infant the onset of sweating is delayed for one to several days [1,30]. Sweating begins first on the face, then later on the palms and remainder of the body. Restriction of sweating does not appear to be related to structural immaturity of the gland or duct but rather to maturity of its autonomic (sympathetic) control [31,32]. Complete neural control of the eccrine sweat gland is not considered to be intact until age 2 or 3 when complexity of the functional sweating activity is equivalent

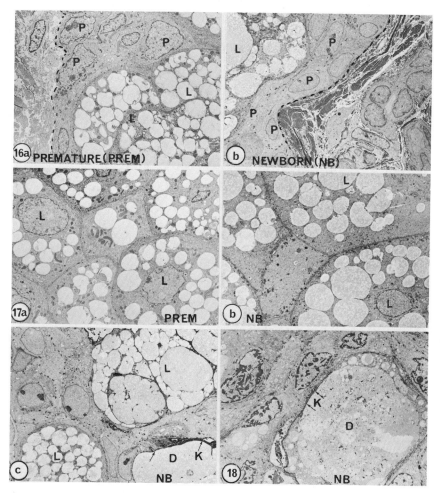

Figures 16, 17, and 18 Sebaceous glands from the skin of a premature and newborn infant. A zone of mitotically active cells (P) forms the peripheral cellular border of an acinus (Fig. 16a,b). Most of the cytoplasm of lipogenic cells (L) is filled with smooth endoplasmic reticulum and droplets (Fig. 17a,b). Centrally, lipid vesicles coalesce (Fig. 17c) and are secreted via a keratinized duct (D) (Figs. 17c and 18). Cells of the proximal sebaceous duct still secrete sebum and are partially keratinized (K) (16a, X 2600; 16b, X 2000; 17a, X 2750; 17b, X 2550; 17c, X 1950 (micrograph courtesy of C. Foster); 18, X 3000).

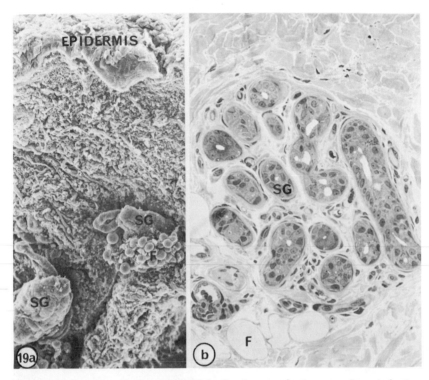

Figure 19 Eccrine sweat glands (SG) in the dermis of a term newborn infant are identical in structure to adult. Several coils of the secretory end piece and terminal segment of the duct lie at the mid- to deep dermis, surrounded by fat (F), capillaries, and unmyelinated nerves (a, X 150; b, X 250).

to that of the adult [1]. Eccrine sweat gland quiescence in the newborn is among the factors which account for the 30% lower transepidermal water loss from newborn skin [2] compared with adult. The density of sweat glands in the skin is greatest at birth as no new glands are formed de novo thereafter.

In both the term newborn and adult the sweat glands were equivalent in size, structural maturity, and position within the dermis (Fig. 19a,b). The level of the gland within the dermis was regionally variable (Fig. 1); depending upon the position, multiple coils of the gland were embedded in fat and surrounded by unmyelinated nerves, a network of capillaries, and a delicate connective tissue mesh. A dense, consistently thick layer of collagen fibrils surrounded the secretory coil and sweat duct in the basal coil (Fig. 20). Three cell types were recog-

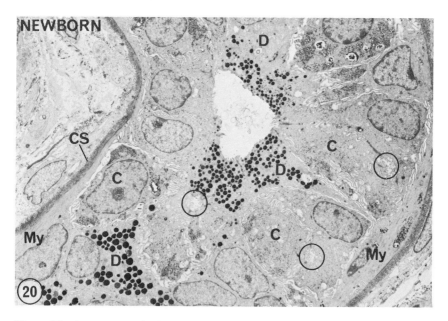

Figure 20 Secretory coil of an eccrine sweat gland in term newborn skin. Dark cells (D) are distinguished by electron-dense granules in the apical cytoplasm. Clear cells (C) contain glycogen. Note the intercellular canaliculi between adjacent clear cells (circled). Myoepithelial cells (My) are evident at the margin of the gland. A thick collagen (CS) sheath encases this tubular gland (× 2600).

nized within the secretory portion of the gland. Two of these, the dark cells and the clear cells, bordered the central lumen and were present in approximately equal numbers. The dark cells are mucigenic cells conspicuous in both histologic preparations and thin sections by the presence of dark-staining, mucin granules in the apical cytoplasm bordering the lumen (Fig. 20). Clear cells are serous-secreting cells that produce most of the sweat. These cells normally contain glycogen deposits unless the gland has been stressed by prolonged periods of sweating. Clear cells interlace with one another and other adjacent cells by means of folded cell borders and long microvilli (Fig. 20). Intercellular canaliculi form between pairs of adjacent clear cells to convey sweat to the lumen of the gland. The boundaries between cells at the canaliculi are sealed by junctional complexes (Fig. 20). The third cell type, the myoepithelial cell, has structural features similar to smooth muscle cells, bundles of banded myofilaments, glycogen and dense plaques spaced at intervals beneath the plasma membrane (Fig. 20).

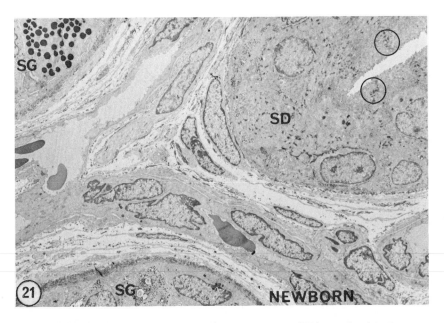

Figure 21 Cross-section of an intradermal sweat duct (SD) proximal to two secretory segments (SG). Three layers of cells form the wall of the duct. Luminal cells are joined by multiple desmosomes (circled) and have a band of keratin filaments at the surface (× 2500).

One-third to one-half of the terminal coil is sweat duct. This structure consists of two to three layers of concentrically arranged cells that are joined at frequent intervals by desmosomes (Fig. 21). Cells of the duct in this region may produce sweat but have a more major functional role in reabsorption of sodium from sweat produced by the secretory segment. Luminal cells have a broad zone of keratin filaments beneath the microvillous border lining the duct (Figs. 21 and 22). Ductile basal cells contain abundant glycogen and large numbers of mitochondria. The pathway of the duct toward the epidermis is a helical "three dimensional meander" [33] that may be seen in the light and scanning electron micrographs of Figures 1 and 23a. As the duct approaches the epidermis, the lumen widens and the bordering cells synthesize a globular form of keratohyalin and undergo a form of incomplete keratinization (Fig. 22a-d). The sweat pore is reinforced by several layers of keratinized squames modified from the epidermal surface (Fig. 22d).

In many respects the sweat glands of the premature infant were more typical

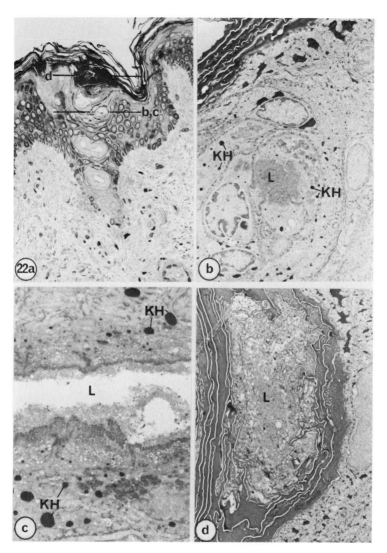

Figure 22 Intraepidermal portions of the sweat duct. The section (a) cuts through helical twists of the duct at several levels. Globular keratohyalin (KH) is seen in the cells that border the duct (b and c). The lumen (L) is filled with membrane vesicles. Microvilli are reinforced with keratin filaments (c). The sweat pore at the surface is surrounded by several layers of keratinized cells (d) (a, × 190, b, × 3600, c, × 5900 (micrograph courtesy of C. Foster); d, × 4000).

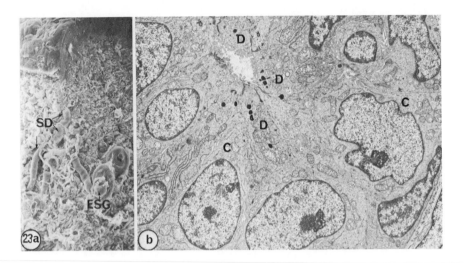

Figure 23 (a) Scanning electron micrograph showing a terminal coil of an eccrine sweat gland (ESG) and duct (SD) in the skin of a premature infant. Note the few coils of the gland (X 90). (b) Secretory cells and eccrine sweat gland from a premature baby. Dark cells (D) have few mucus granules. Clear cells (C) show little evidence of differentiation (X 4200).

of the fetal state than the adult; end-pieces were limited to a few turns of the coil (Fig. 23a) and cells within the secretory regions were less fully differentiated. Mucigenic dark cells were distinguished from others only by the presence of a few mucin granules in the apical cytoplasm. Clear cells lacked the distinctive microvillous borders and intercellular canaliculi (Fig. 23b). Minimal numbers of myofilaments were observed in the cytoplasm of myoepithelial cells. Sweat ducts were fully formed and patent. Our observations of relatively undifferentiated cells within the secretory end portion of the gland suggest that it is questionable whether the gland is "morphologically mature" [1] by 28 weeks; studies in which the functional competence of these glands in the premature baby has been tested have shown the sweating response to be absent or limited and are therefore in accord with the morphological interpretation [32,34,35].

Nerves and Vessels

The architecture of the nerve and vascular networks alike develop early in the fetus but organize into adult patterns only after the first few months of post-natal life; these systems, like nearly all other properties of the skin, also exhibit considerable regional variation.

Typically, the vessels which supply the skin are organized into subpapillary and deep reticular horizontal plexuses interconnected by vertical arcades of vessels and from which extend elements of the microcirculation. Special vascular networks surround hair follicles and glands of the skin. Venous plexuses roughly parallel the arterial distribution. Arterial-venous anastomoses are common in mature skin. The arterial and venous patterns become established in the seventh month of fetal life and are influenced by the surrounding tissue, hence modified in different parts of the body depending upon the structure of the skin, the mechanical pressures, and the function of the skin in that particular region [36].

At birth, the subpapillary plexus is disorganized. A rich, anastomosing network of capillaries lies in the upper dermis and imparts the characteristic red color to the newborn. The vastness of this and other capillary networks diminishes in the first weeks with the loss of lanugo hairs, reduced activity of sebaceous glands, and increased skin surface area [37,38]. Except for the palms, soles, and nail folds, no papillary loops project toward the epidermis before the first week. Between weeks 4 and 5, papillary loops are seen in all areas and are well-established between the 14th and 17th weeks. The less random, adultlike pattern is acquired as skin growth slows down; the greatest rate of skin growth occurs during the first 2 weeks after birth, then proceeds more slowly until the third month when the adult vascular patterns can be recognized [38]. In general, however, the maturity of the vascular pattern depends more upon the structure of the particular tissue than the age from birth [37]. Other physiological properties of the cardiovascular system influence formation of different elements of the cutaneous vasculature after birth, including low blood pressure, elevated blood viscosity and extravasation through the vessel wall, decreased oxygen tension, decreased sedimentation rate, and decreased red cell flexibility [37,38].

There is no adequate way to demonstrate these features in routine histological preparations and thin sectioned specimens, although a comparison of the vascular networks can be made on a superficial basis among the body regions from the photomicrographs of Figure 1.

The nervous network in the newborn, like the vascular network, also has a more random structural organization than in the adult and is functionally less mature as measured by the axon reflex reaction (flare reaction to histamine). That a term newborn infant can respond to histamine implies that the components of the reflex arc are assembled and have functional capability, but the high stimulus threshold necessary to elicit the response suggests that the smooth muscle of the vessel may be less responsive to the stimulus or that the vasoconstrictor tone may be greater than in the adult [39]. An even poorer axon flare response is characteristic for the premature infant weighing less than 1400 g [39]. Maturity of the peripheral nervous system, therefore, is a function of gestational age and weight more than age as measured from birth [1]. It is the view of many [40,41] that cutaneous nerves continue to develop until puberty or beyond.

On a structural basis, most of the nerves identified in premature and term newborn skin were small diameter, unmyelinated, sensory and autonomic nerves. Unmyelinated nerves in the premature infant were characteristically fetal in structure [42]; large numbers of axons were enclosed within Schwann cells (Fig. 24a,b), often clustered in axonal bundles that shared a common chamber within the Schwann cell wrapping. With increasing age fewer axons and axonal bundles remained within one Schwann cell; correspondingly, an increase in myelinated fibers was observed (compare Figs. 24 and 25) [43,44]. Unmyelinated nerves in term newborn skin typically contained more axons within a single Schwann cell than an adult nerve found in a similar location within the dermis, but fewer than characteristically seen in the premature skin. Small axonal bundles also were seen in these samples but were not common and contained no more than two to three grouped axons (Fig. 25). Multiaxonal bundles were reported in the newborn skin at the site of an adnexal polyp [42]. Larger-diameter nerves which contained a combination of myelinated and unmyelinated fibers were restricted primarily to the deeper regions of the dermis.

Specialized sensory receptors are developed to varying degrees at birth. Pacinian corpuscles are abundant in hairless areas of the hands and feet and fully developed in structure. From this point, a substantial number are lost and those remaining are remodelled [45] (Fig. 26). Merkel's corpuscles of the digital skin begin to diminish in number and become restricted in position even before birth or shortly thereafter. By contrast, Meissner's touch receptors are not fully formed at birth. These structures continue to undergo morphological changes in such a characteristic sequence that the state of the receptor at any given time has predictive value for determining age [45]. Free nerve endings undergo fewer changes in structure from birth to old age.

COMMENT

From this survey of the histological and ultrastructural properties of newborn skin in comparison with adult and premature infant skin, it may be concluded that, in the newborn, the epidermis and epidermal appendages are nearly identical with their counterpart adult structures. On the other hand, the dermis shares features in common with both premature and adult skin, and in a sense may exemplify a transitional state between the two age/structure groups. The total thickness of the dermis is less than that of the adult. Collagenous fiber bundles of the reticular dermis, in particular, are smaller than those of the adult; elastic fibers are immature. The vascular and nervous networks are disorganized at birth and undergo substantial reorganization depending upon the surrounding

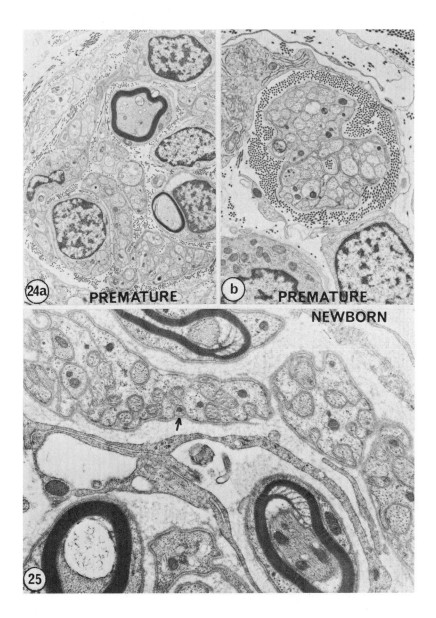

Figures 24 and 25 Nerves in the papillary dermis from a premature (Fig. 24) and term (Fig. 25) newborn. Unmyelinated nerves with large numbers of axons are within a single Schwann cell; bundles of grouped axons lie within a single infolding of the Schwann cell in the premature newborn (Fig. 24b). Axon bundles are less common in unmyelinated nerves of the term newborn and usually include only two to three axons (Fig. 25, arrow) (24a, × 5300; 24b, × 10,200; 25, × 17,000).

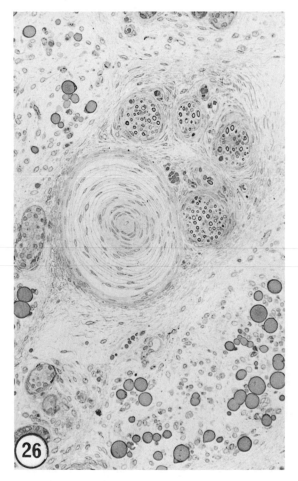

Figure 26 Morphologically mature Pacinian corpuscle in the skin of the finger from a full-term newborn (X 90).

tissue and rate of growth of the skin. Nonetheless, structure of all layers of the epidermis, characteristics of the dermis, density and size of the appendages, and architecture of the microcirculatory and nerve networks reflect the site from which the sample was obtained. Thus, regional variation in the development and organization of all cutaneous structures is expressed well before birth and is as remarkable in the newborn as it is in the adult.

ACKNOWLEDGMENT

This work was supported by USPHS Grants AM-21577 and AM-07019 from the National Institutes of Health. The author wishes to thank Ms. Doris Ringer for expert preparation of the manuscript.

REFERENCES

1. Solomon LM, Esterly NB: Neonatal dermatology. I. The newborn skin. J Pediatr 77:888-894, 1970.
2. Wildnauer RH, Kennedy R: Transepidermal water loss of human newborns. J Invest Dermatol 54:483-486 (1970).
3. Solomon LM, Esterly NB: Structure of fetal and neonatal skin, in *Major Problems in Clinical Pediatrics, Vol IX*, edited by Schaffer Alexander J. Saunders, Philadelphia, 1973, pp 1-16.
4. Solomon LM, Esterly NB: Functional components of the skin, in *Major Problems in Clinical Pediatrics, Vol IX*, edited by Schaffer Alexander J. Saunders, Philadelphia, 1973, pp 17-22.
5. Beare JM, Rook A: The newborn, in *Textbook of Dermatology*, edited by Rook A, Wilkinson DS, Ebling FJG. Blackwell, Oxford, 1958, pp 112-114.
6. Karnovsky MJ: A formaldehyde-glutaraldehyde fixative of high osmolarity for use in electron microscopy. J Cell Biol 27:137A, 1965.
7. Luft JH: Improvements in epoxy resin embedding. J Biophys Biochem Cytol 9:409-414, 1961.
8. Cohen AL, Marlow DP, Garner GE: A rapid critical point method using fluorocarbons ("Freons") as intermediate and transitional fluids. J Microsc 7:331-342, 1968.
9. Hutchinson-Smith B: Skinfold thickness in infancy in relation to birth-weight. Dev Med Child Neurol 15:628-634, 1973.
10. Montagna W: An introduction to sebaceous glands. J Invest Dermatol 62:120-123, 1974.
11. Fujita H, Asagami C, Murota S, Murozumi S: Ultrastructural study of embryonic sebaceous cells, especially of their sebum droplet formation. Acta Derm Venereol (Stockh) 52:99-115, 1972.
12. Ramasatry P, Downing DT, Pochi PE, Strauss JS: Chemical composition of human skin surface lipids from birth to puberty. J Invest Dermatol 54:139-144, 1970.
13. Kürkkäinen J, Nikkari T, Ruponen S, Haahti E: Lipids of the vernix caseosa. J Invest Dermatol 44:333-338, 1965.
14. Nazzaro-Porro M, Passi S, Boniforti L, Belsito F: Effects of aging on fatty acids in skin surface lipids. J Invest Dermatol 73:112-117, 1979.
15. Plewig G: Regional differences in cell sizes in the human stratum corneum. Part II. Effects of sex and age. J Invest Dermatol 54:19-20, 1970.

16. Becker SW, Zimmerman AA: Further studies on melanocytes and melanogenesis in the human fetus and newborn. J Invest Dermatol 25:103-112, 1955.

17. Hamada H: Changes in melanocyte distribution of the normal human epidermis according to age. Jpn J Dermatol 82:223-232, 1972.

18. Nachman RL, Esterly NB: Increased skin permeability in preterm infants. J Pediatr 79:628-632, 1971.

19. Hashimoto I, Anton-Lamprecht I, Meyburg P: Epidermolysis bullosa hereditaria letalis: report of a case and probable ultrastructural defects. Helv Pediatr Acta 30:543-552, 1976.

20. Briggaman RA, Wheeler CE Jr: Epidermolysis bullosa dystrophica-recessive: a possible role of anchoring fibrils in the pathogenesis. J Invest Dermatol 65:203-211, 1975.

21. Cotta-Pereira G, Rodrigo FG, Bittencourt-Sampaio S: Oxytalan, elaunin, and elastic fibers in the human skin. J Invest Dermatol 66:143-148, 1976.

22. Deutsch TA, Esterly NB: Elastic fibers in fetal dermis. J Invest Dermatol 65:320-323, 1975.

23. Spicer SS, Brissie RM, Thompson NT: Variability of dermal elastin visualized ultrastructurally with iron hematoxylin. Am J Pathol 79:481-498, 1975.

24. Berger HM, King J, Doughty S, Wharton BA: Nutrition, sex, gestational age and hair growth in babies. Arch Dis Child 53:290-294, 1978.

25. Montagna W: General review of the anatomy, growth, and development of hair in man, in *Biology and Disease of the Hair*, edited by Toda K. University Park Press, Baltimore, 1976, pp xxi-xxxi.

26. Barman JM, Pecoraro V, Astore I, Ferrer J: The first stage in the natural history of the human scalp hair cycle. J Invest Dermatol 48:138-142, 1967.

27. Pecoraro V, Astore I, Barman JM: Cycle of scalp hair of the newborn child. J Invest Dermatol 43:145-147, 1964.

28. Nasseem Husain OA, Sinclair L: Studies on the cytology of amniotic fluid and of the newborn infant's skin in relation to maturity of the infant. Proc R Soc Med 64:1213-1217, 1971.

29. Hashimoto K, Gross BG, Lever WF: The ultrastructure of the skin of human embryos I. The intraepidermal eccrine sweat duct. J Invest Dermatol 45:139-151, 1965.

30. Brück K: Temperature regulation in the newborn infant. Biol Neonat 3:65-119, 1961.

31. Behrendt H, Green M: Nature of the sweating deficit of prematurely born neonates. Observations on babies with the heroin withdrawal syndrome. N Engl J Med 286:1376-1379, 1972.

32. Foster KG, Hey EN, Katz G: The response of the sweat glands of the newborn baby to thermal stimuli and to intradermal acetylcholine. J Physiol (Lond) 203:B-29, 1969.

33. Wells TR, Landing BH: The helical course of the human eccrine sweat duct. J Invest Dermatol 51:177-185, 1968.

34. Sinclair JC: Thermal control in premature infants. Annu Rev Med 23:129-148, 1972.
35. Green M, Behrendt H: Sweating capacity of neonates. Am J Dis Child 118:725-732, 1969.
36. Korneva NA: Local structural characteristics of the human skin and architecture of its capillary bed. Arkh Anat Gistol Embriol 56:64-70, 1969.
37. Ryan TJ: Structure, pattern and shape of the blood vessels of the skin, in *The Physiology and Pathophysiology of the Skin, Vol 2*, edited by Jarrett A. Academic Press, New York, 1973, pp 577-651.
38. Perera P, Kurban AK, Ryan TJ: The development of the cutaneous microvascular system in the newborn. Br J Dermatol 82 (Suppl 5):86-91, 1970.
39. Wilkes T, Freedman RI, Hodgman J, Levan NE: The sensitivity of the axon reflex in term and premature infants. J Invest Dermatol 47:491-492, 1966.
40. Winkelmann RK: Cutaneous nerves, in *Ultrastructure of Normal and Abnormal Skin*, edited by Zelickson AS. Lea & Febiger, Philadelphia, 1967, pp 202-2237.
41. Sinclair D: Normal anatomy of sensory nerves and receptors, in *The Physiology and Pathophysiology of the Skin, Vol 2*, edited by Jarrett A. Academic Press, New York, 1973, pp 348-402.
42. Sato S, Ogihara Y, Higara K, Nishijima A, Hidano A: Fine structure of unmyelinated nerves in neonatal skin. J Cutan Pathol 4:1-8, 1977.
43. Gamble HJ, Breathnach AS: An electron microscope study of human foetal peripheral nerves. J Anat 99:573-584, 1965.
44. Gamble HJ: Further electron microscope studies of human foetal peripheral nerves. J Anat 100:487-502, 1966.
45. Cauna K: The effect of aging on the receptor organs of the human dermis, in *Advances in Biology of Skin, Vol 1*, edited by Montagna W. Pergamon Press, Oxford, 1960, pp 63-93.

APPENDAGES

2

Comparison of Adult and Neonatal Skin Eccrine Sweating

MARVIN GREEN

State University of New York, Stony Brook, New York

Although most concern about newborns' competence in thermoregulation relates to the ability to conserve heat, they also appear to be handicapped in the facility with which hyperthermia is prevented. The major reason for this difficulty is impairment of the ability to dissipate heat from the body by sweating. That the apparently mature newborn has not yet attained full development of sweating function has long been assumed by pediatricians. Not only is generalized sweating unusual in healthy infants born at term, but it appears to be totally lacking in the premature baby. Concrete evidence to substantiate this impression has been developed over more than 30 years. Information elucidating the precise reasons for the neonatal handicap in sweating has only recently been developed. The fact that the newborn is comparatively resistant to sweating in response to environmental temperature can be verified from studies on adults and newborns. Women exposed to warm environmental temperature begin to show sweat secretion at 32°C, while the thermal threshold for men is only 29°C [1]. In contrast, Uchino [2] failed to evoke sweating in neonates on the first day of life in spite of exposure to an environmental temperature range of 33-42°C. The advent of sweating ranged from the second to the 18th day of life. For a group of nine premature infants between 34 and 37 weeks of gestational age, sweating responsiveness occurred distinctly later than for the mature infant; in one sweating was not observed for 3 weeks and in another it was not yet evident at 33 days of age. In

Dedicated to the memory of Hans Behrendt, my mentor, colleague, and dear friend.

subsequent studies it has been shown that neonatal sweating could be evoked more regularly if environmental temperature was sufficiently intense to increase rectal temperature to more than 37.5°C, an environmental temperature of 36-37°C being needed to effect such elevations of rectal temperature. Most infants born within 3 weeks prior to term were capable of sweating, while babies between 34 and 37 weeks of postconceptional age were less capable of sweating. In this latter group of infants the ability to produce sweat in response to environmental thermal stimulation was rapidly facilitated with increasing postnatal age, a significantly higher proportion showing sweating by 2 weeks after birth. Infants of less than 30 weeks of postconceptional age were incapable of sweating even when rectal temperature was increased to 37.8°C. Regional differences in sweating onset were also noted. In more prematurely born infants, sweating tended to appear initially on the limbs, and in those of greater maturity sweating first appeared on the forehead and temple, later on the chest, and finally on the legs [3].

On the basis of such evidence the clinical impression that newborns fail to show sweating in their natural environment appears to be substantiated; however, the precise reasons for neonatal refractoriness to sweating remained unclear. It appeared reasonable that this might be clarified by investigating the functional competence of the sweating apparatus, i.e., sweat gland, sudomotor nerve, and sudorific centers. This chapter is primarily devoted to the roles of each of these components in neonatal sweating and compares their functional capacity with that previously established for the adult.

TESTS OF SWEAT GLAND FUNCTION

The total number of eccrine sweat glands is completed before birth; at that time their density is greater than later in life, due to the increase in surface area of the skin with growth [4]. The variation in concentration of functional sweat glands at different age ranges must be taken into consideration in evaluating the comparative secretory efficacy of eccrine sweat glands in neonates and adults. During the first 2½ years of life a lower proportion of these glands exhibit secretory activity [5]. Such comparisons may also be impeded by the continued existence of obstructed secretory coils in babies who are born prematurely, since vacuolization of the central column of epithelial cells with the formation of a continuous hollow channel may not be completed until the end of the seventh fetal month [6], preventing emission of sweat from the ducts. In either circumstance, the amount of sweat produced in a precise area of skin must be corrected for density of sweat glands and expressed as rate of secretion per gland.

Local responsiveness of the sweat gland has been elicited by a variety of pharmacological agents administered in minute dosage either intradermally or by iontophoresis. Locally applied heat can also evoke sweat gland responses limited to the site of stimulation. In addition to a direct glandular effect of heat, neural transmission is also involved in determining the ability of the sweat gland to respond [7,8].

Because of the cited difficulties in comparing localized sweat production quantitatively in adults and neonates, the preferred method would appear to be the determination of the minimally effective stimulus capable of evoking a localized sweating response (threshold). For sudorific drugs, consecutive 10-fold serial dilutions with 0.9% NaCl can be prepared (w/v) and given intradermally by means of a tuberculin syringe. This form of local administration is superior to iontophoresis since the amount of drug absorbed by the latter method cannot be accurately determined. To avoid the possible confounding effect of regional differences in sweating activity [3] identical skin regions should be compared, the volar aspect of the forearm being suitable.

The ambient temperature should be lower than that capable of evoking generalized sweating reactions. In this regard, one must be cognizant of the different thermal thresholds for generalized sweating in adults and neonates [1,2,9]. Although comparative studies at the neutral thermal range might be warranted, unfortunately this differs for adults and neonates. For the neonate the neutral thermal range, 32-34°C [9] supercedes the threshold for generalized sweating in adults. Therefore a reasonable solution might be the selection of ambient temperatures unlikely to evoke generalized sweating. This would appear justified by observations that sweat gland activity on a particular body area is more likely to be influenced by local skin temperature than environmental temperature [8, 10,11]. Therefore testing of skin sites with equivalent temperature would appear more appropriate. Visualization of sweating can easily be established by a variety of colorimetric reactions; of these the starch-iodine reaction is the most commonly used.

Response to Acetylcholine and Adrenaline

Intradermally administered acetylcholine stimulates the sweat gland much as its physiologic equivalent does when emitted at sudomotor nerve endings. In evaluating local responses to exogenous acetylcholine we must consider those responses indicative of this local action and exclude those due to the sudomotor axon reflex which may also be induced by this drug. The local sudorific effect of acetylcholine can be inhibited by atropine and enhanced by cholinesterase inhibitors [12,13], indicating that the local sweating reaction to exogenous acetylcholine is the counterpart of physiologic sweating.

Although intradermally administered adrenergic drugs can also produce local sweating [14-16], generalized sweating is not likely to occur following systemic administration of adrenergic agents, and physiologic sweating is not believed to have an adrenergic component. Patients with pheochromocytomas, however, may have hyperhidrosis. Tending to confirm the absence of a role in normal sweating is the absence of an inhibitory effect by atropine on local adrenergic sweating [14,16,17]. These sweating reactions are inhibited by adrenergic blocking agents [14,16,17]. Because of the long duration of sweating responses it is unlikely that the explanation for the effect of adrenergic stimulation is the expulsion of preformed sweat by contraction of myoepithelial cells surrounding the ducts [18]. A hypothetical explanation for the effectiveness of intracutaneous adrenergic agents is the existence of specific sweat gland receptors distinct from cholinergic receptors. What remains unexplained is the role of these putative receptors in natural sweating.

The reactivity of the eccrine sweat gland to local stimulation with adrenaline varies with age [15]. In the second and third decades concentrations as low as 10^{-7} can produce sweating. In younger children and in adults aged 60-70 years the sweating threshold is higher and concentrations more dilute than 10^{-4} are ineffective.

Local sweating thresholds have been determined for acetylcholine and adrenaline in 15 low-birth-weight (14 premature) and 14 full-size (13 mature) newborns during the first 7 days of life by Behrendt and Green [19]. Tests were carried out with all infants placed in incubators set at 30°C. Abdominal skin temperature, temperature on the volar surface of the forearm (test site), and core temperature were measured by thermistors. Arithmetic means for skin temperatures were almost identical for both groups; the average core temperature was 0.6°C lower in the low-birth-weight neonates than the full-size neonates. The test site was prepared with a 2% solution of iodine in 95% ethyl alcohol. When dry, 0.01-0.02 ml of one of a series of 10-fold dilutions, 10^{-3}-10^{-7} (w/v), of acetylcholine or adrenaline was given by means of a tuberculin syringe fitted with a 26 or 27 gauge needle, the minimally effective concentration being determined. The site was coated with a 50% suspension of corn starch in castor oil to prevent evaporation of sweat [15]. The presence of sweat droplets was shown by the local appearance of at least four blue-purple spots appearing within 25 min. These could be seen easily with a five-power magnifying lens; larger droplets could be detected without this. A control injection of 0.9% NaCl was given in the contralateral forearm. Although the diluent failed to produce sweating responses, the simultaneous appearance of sweating at both sites signalled the presence of generalized sweating, so-called background sweating (Fig. 1), which invalidated the test. Only the sweating response due to the muscarinic action of acetylcholine was considered to be positive; it began within 3 min and reached its maximum at 5-20 min (Fig. 2). Responses to adrenaline appeared at 1-3 min surrounding the injection site; the reaction then spread to the blanched pseudopods produced by the vasoconstrictor effect of adrenaline on the local lymphatic channels (Fig. 3). The reaction often failed to reach its maximum as long as 25 min after

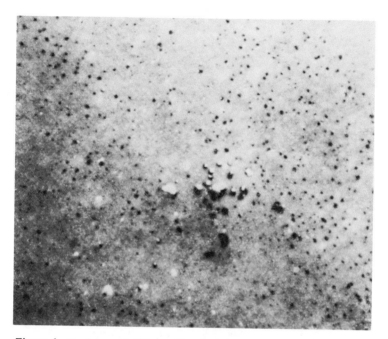

Figure 1 Background (Thermal) sweating in a full-size 4-day-old infant tested with acetylcholine. Generalized sweating obscures the local sweating response to the drug. (*Source*: From Behrendt H, Green M: Am J Dis Child 117:299–306, 1969. Copyright 1969, American Medical Association.)

administration. Positive reactions were obtained with each drug in all 14 full-size neonates. Of the 15 low-birth-weight infants, 13 failed to react to the greatest concentration of acetylcholine and eight failed to respond to the maximal concentration of adrenaline. For both acetylcholine and adrenaline, the proportion of subjects with thresholds between 10^{-4} and 10^{-7} was significantly greater in full-size than low-birth-weight infants with the difference between the positive thresholds in this range being much higher than the lower confidence limit for a coefficient of confidence of 0.95, chi-square = 5.991, with two degrees of freedom. Differences in sweating thresholds are even more pronounced when related to gestational age. Sweating thresholds for all subjects, arranged by gestational age, are shown in Figure 4. Sweat gland reactivity failed to be shown with the strongest concentrations of acetylcholine and adrenaline used in most neonates less than 36 weeks of gestation; however one infant of only 32 weeks of gestation exhibited a positive response to adrenaline 10^{-3}.

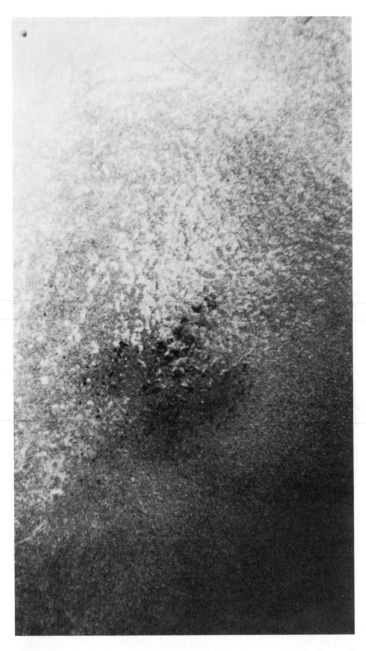

Figure 2 Local muscarinic sweating response to acetylcholine. (*Source*: from Behrendt H, Green M: Am J Dis Child 117:299-306, 1969. Copyright 1969, American Medical Association.)

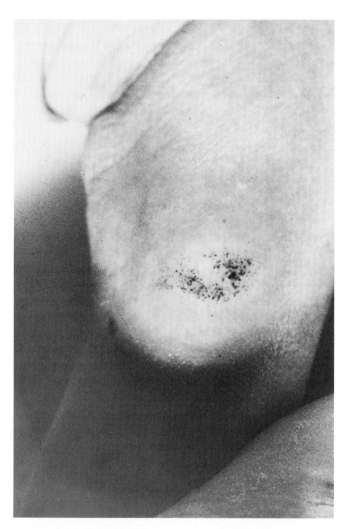

Figure 3 Local sweating response to adrenaline. (*Source*: from Behrendt H, Green M: Am J Dis Child 117:299-306, 1969. Copyright 1969, American Medical Association.)

In follow-up observations on 11 premature infants who initially failed to show local sweating responses to single concentrations of acetylcholine 10^{-5} or adrenaline 10^{-4}, positive reactions were elicited later in seven at an age range of 4-38 days, while four continued to show unresponsive sweat glands at 11-39 days of

Concentration

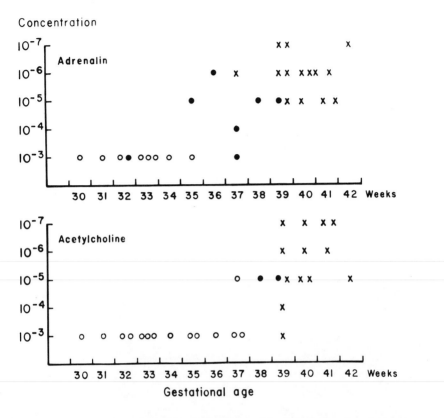

Figure 4 Sweating thresholds for adrenaline and acetylcholine in relation to gestational age in 29 neonates. ○, negative response 10^{-3} concentration; ●, threshold concentration in low-birth-weight infant; X, threshold concentration in full-size infant. (*Source*: from Behrendt H, Green M: Am J Dis Child 117:209-306, 1969. Copyright 1969, American Medical Association.)

age. There was no obvious relationship between the age of onset of sweating and the degree of prematurity nor were significant differences shown between male and female newborns.

Since both adrenaline and acetylcholine exert their effect by acting directly on sweat glands [12,13,15-17] the demonstration of positive reactions in mature neonates indicates that function of the end-organ is intact and shows responsiveness of a similar order as the adult. This is certainly so for adrenaline [16]. Because the weakest dilution of acetylcholine was not as low as that found to be effective in adults it is not known whether the mature neonate can show sweating responsiveness to acetylcholine 10^{-12} [20]. The lack of reactivity of the sweat gland of the premature infant born at 34 weeks and less suggests the presence of a temporary block in the receptor mechanism of secretory cells. Since generalized thermal sweating can be facilitated by duration of postnatal age in infants born prematurely [3], refractoriness of the sweat gland to local stimulation may also be enhanced by postnatal age; however, I am not aware that this has been demonstrated thus far.

We had planned initially to test premature and term subjects at an environmental temperature of 32°C, approximating thermoneutrality. Surprisingly, a number of mature neonates showed generalized sweating at this temperature, necessitating the adoption of the lower temperature used. The influence of environmental temperature on local sweating responsiveness to drugs is less important than temperature on the test site [8,10,11]; the presence of equivalent temperature at this location for our subjects would appear to weigh more heavily in accounting for our results than dissimilar tolerance for environmental thermal stimulation by premature and mature infants.

Evidence for Alpha- and Beta-Adrenergic Receptors

Other adrenergic agents besides adrenaline are capable of evoking local sweat gland responsiveness. Both norepinephrine and isoproterenol [21] have this effect, although their effectiveness tends to be less than that of adrenaline. Since the sympathomimetic effects of isoproterenol are predominantly those of beta-receptor stimulation, while those of adrenaline and norepinephrine are principally those of alpha-receptor stimulation, the elicitation of distinctive sweating responses for these drugs might indicate the existence of alpha and beta sweat gland receptors. In this regard, an interesting finding distinguishing local sweating responsiveness to adrenaline and isoproterenol is worth noting. Although the principal effect of adrenaline is to cause local sweating responses, less well known is the inhibitory response of adrenaline administered by iontophoresis or intradermally [22] immediately prior to generalized sweating provoked by increased environmental temperature. Wada et al. [23] have also demonstrated inhibition of the sudomotor axon reflex by preliminary injection of adrenaline in the test area.

Behrendt and Green [24] carried out the following tests to determine the comparative effects of adrenaline and isoproterenol on local inhibition of sweating (sparing effect). A dose of adrenaline of 0.004-0.005 mg or isoproterenol 0.005 mg exceeding the threshold for sweating and contained in 0.02 ml of 0.9% NaCl solution was given intradermally into the volar surface of the forearm. Following this, 6 ml of 0.2% aqueous solution of pilocarpine nitrate was iontophoresed for 4 min at 2 mA into a 4 × 5 cm superimposed area with the injection site at its center. Sweating was permitted for 10 min under a transparent plastic cover. Upon removal, the skin was rinsed and dried with gauze, and the entire area was painted with Wada's reagents [15] to visualize sweat droplets during the ensuing 15 min. In each of five subjects ranging in age from 18 months to 42 years an inhibitory effect of adrenaline on pilocarpine-induced local sweating was clearly demonstrable. Around the injection site was an area free or almost totally free of sweat spots surrounded by a dense sweating reaction to pilocarpine. For five subjects ranging in age from 3½ months to 9 years given isoproterenol, sweat droplets were uniformly dispersed throughout the test site. The differential reactions are shown in the sweat prints, Figures 5 and 6.

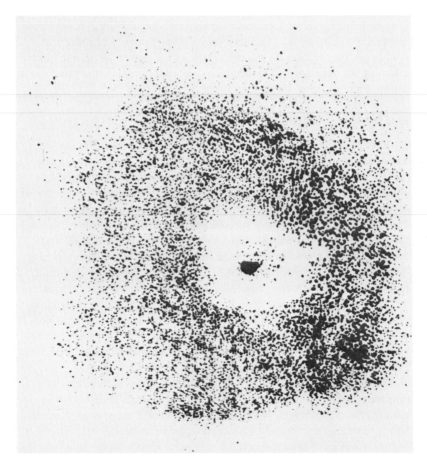

Figure 5 Inhibitory effect of intradermal injection of adrenaline on sweating produced by pilocarpine iontophoresis (alpha-adrenergic receptor?).

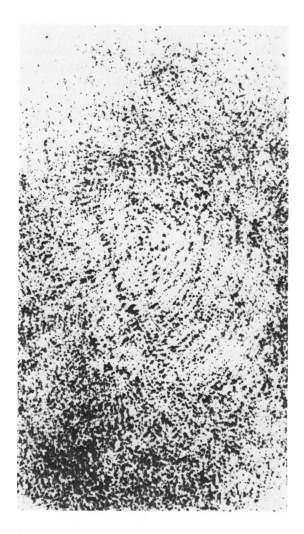

Figure 6 Effect of intradermal injection of isoproterenol on sweating produced by pilocarpine iontophoresis (beta-adrenergic receptor?).

In 11 children ranging in age from 2 days to 12 years who showed background sweating during the course of threshold determinations with adrenaline, the sparing effect was observed in five. There were no significant differences between doses of adrenaline that inhibited sweating and those that failed to exert this effect.

Although speculation about the differential effects of adrenaline and isopro-terenol on local sweat gland inhibition may warrant consideration of distinct alpha and beta sweat gland receptors, absence of physiologic adrenergic sweating and lack of sweating responsiveness to otherwise systemically effective doses of adrenergic agents tend to cast doubt on their existence. Gibson [25] suggests a reasonable alternative explanation for local adrenergic inhibition of sweating. He believes that the sparing effect is actually due to alpha-adrenergic vasoconstric-tion which is presumed to impede diffusion of adrenaline to the immediate prox-imity of the sweat gland. His explanation for the sparing effect notwithstanding, Gibson also provides substantive evidence for the presence of alpha- and beta-adrenergic receptors on sweat glands. He found that iontophoresis of equivalent amounts of atropine failed to block local sweating reactions produced by intra-dermally administered norepinephrine but effectively blocked isoproterenol in-duced sweating both in patients with cystic fibrosis and in controls [26].

Some additional recent observations fail to clarify if there is a physiologic counterpart for localized adrenergic sweating. Although cholinesterase abounds in the nerve fibers in proximity to the eccrine sweat glands of humans [27], re-cently Uno and Montagna have demonstrated the existence of catecholamine-containing nerve terminals in the vicinity of eccrine sweat glands in Macaques [28]. The results of studies with the alpha-adrenergic antagonist phentolamine have only served to confuse the issue. Not only can it effectively block the sweat-ing response to alpha-adrenergic drugs, but it also has been shown to be capable of inhibiting local cholinergic sweating [29].

The Cholinergic Receptor

Although comparative efficacy of the sweat gland receptor to stimulation with exogenous acetylcholine has been defined in adults and neonates, determination of the ability of the neurohumoral transmitter to effect sweating in vivo has special requirements. It requires an assessment of the competence of the terminal sudomotor rami to elaborate this compound as well as its ability to disseminate to a responsive sweat gland. This portion of the sweating apparatus can be studied selectively by means of local stimulation tests using cholinesterase inhibitors. These agents permit the accumulation of endogenous acetylcholine by interfering with its degradation to acetic acid and choline. Coon and Rothman [30] have shown that the cholinesterase inhibitor physostigmine greatly potentiated the sweating response produced by intradermal injection of acetylcholine. Janowitz and Gross-man [12] showed that physostigmine as well as neostigmine could produce local sweating responses when given intradermally to adult subjects; however neither they nor others [31] have attempted to define threshold concentrations. Green and Behrendt [32] studied the ability of neostigmine to promote local sweating responses in mature and premature neonates by determining sweating threshold concentrations for this drug. They found that sweating responses could be induced by intradermal injection of 0.01-0.02 ml of 10^{-4}-10^{-7} (w/v) concentrations of this drug in 14 out of 15 full-size neonates and in only four of 17 low-birth-weight babies within the first 8 days after birth. By means of a test of homogeneity the difference in the proportion of newborn infants with thresholds of 10^{-4} or less was significantly greater for full size than low birth weight neonates, $\chi^2 = 6.635$, P < 0.01 with a lower confidence limit of 0.313 and one degree of freedom. Comparisons were made for mature and premature newborns and showed an even more striking difference. The distribution of sweating responses by birth weight and gestation is shown in Figure 7. The local sweating response to neostigmine in the newborn appears more slowly than the local muscarinic effect due to intradermal acetylcholine and is characterized by a less dense but more dispersed response. The evolution of this reaction is consistent with the gradual accumulation of acetylcholine in vivo which ultimately

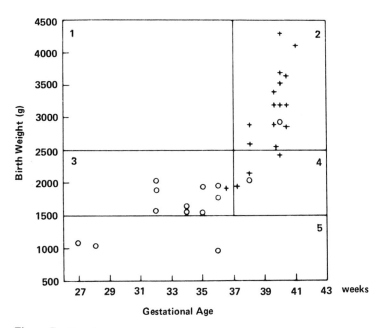

Figure 7 Sweating responses to neostigmine relative to birth weight and gestational age in 32 neonates. +, positive reaction to $\leqslant 10^{-4}$, ○, negative reaction to 10^{-4} (strongest used); field 4, small-for-date infants. (*Source:* from Green M, Behrendt, H: Am J Dis Child 120:434-438, 1970. Copyright 1970, American Medical Association.)

supercedes the endogenous threshold for sweating. In stimulation tests combining equal amounts of subthreshold concentrations of acetylcholine and neostigmine on three full-term and four premature neonates, the mature neonates showed positive sweating reactions while all of the premature infants were unresponsive. Only in the mature infant could we demonstrate the potentiating action of cholinesterase inhibition. Based on the available evidence, the competence of the terminal sudomotor rami to emit acetylcholine and the glandular receptor to respond to it appears to be equivalent for the mature neonate and the adult. However, it is not possible to state whether this portion of the sweating apparatus is undeveloped in the premature infant whose sweat gland is refractory to direct stimulation with either acetylcholine or adrenaline.

That the framework for peripheral neurohumoral transmission is already present for even the least mature infant at the time of birth is shown by the presence of cholinesterase-rich nerves surrounding the sweat gland as early as 4½ months of gestation [27].

TESTS OF COMBINED SWEAT GLAND AND NEURAL FUNCTION

Local Thermal Stimulation of Sweating

The comparison of eccrine sweating in adults and neonates has been addressed by examining the functional competence of the anatomic divisions of the sweating apparatus. In studies devoted to local sweating produced by heat there is not only direct glandular stimulation but a superimposed influence mediated by sudomotor impulses which originate centrally, the precise location of the source not being clearly defined.

Randall [8] exposed adults to radiant heat over a skin area 10-20 mm in diameter. By means of starch-iodine paper prints he was able to detect profuse local sweating which at times persisted for several hours, long after stimulation was ended and skin temperature had returned to normal. The temperature at the test site during heating had ranged from 38.4 to 45.5°C. Even after local iontophoresis of atropine, a diminished sweating reaction could still be produced by heating. In local thermal stimulation tests carried out by Issekutz et al. [7] both at high (29-30°C) and low (18-20°C) environmental temperature, the local sweating response was considerably attenuated in the colder environment. Intradermal injection of procaine prior to thermal stimulation only inhibited the response produced at the higher environmental temperature. They also found that the sudorific effect of local heating was markedly inhibited or prevented by submerging the contralateral arm in cold water of 1-14°C. Evidence for the operation of a neural factor is also provided by the study of Green and Behrendt on children and adults with familial dysautonomia [33]. This disease is characterized by generalized hyperhidrosis presumed to be caused by an increased excitatory state of sweating centers [34]. For these patients, local sweating reactions could be produced with a thermal stimulus no higher than 38.7°C, while for control subjects the minimally effective thermal stimulus was no lower than 40°C. Janowitz and Grossman [12] studied the effect of local heating on denervated sweat glands in adults with lumbar sympathectomies. Sweating responses could be elicited in spite of negative reactions to intradermal adrenaline and acetylcholine. Therefore, it appears that two mechanisms are operative in the production of local sweating reactions in response to stimulation with heat: one a direct glandular component that is not mediated via the cholinergic receptor, and the second a neural component that is mediated via reflex centers and the cholinergic sweat gland receptor. What appears unique is that the area of responsiveness is more or less conterminous with the area of stimulation; therefore the neural component is not that of an axon reflex.

Green and Behrendt [35] performed local thermal stimulation tests with conductive heat in mature and premature neonates within the first 8 days of life. To evaluate the effect of ambient temperature, mature infants were tested at different ranges of environmental temperature. Premature infants were tested in incubators with abdominal skin temperature controlled thermostatically at 36-36.9°C by means of the servo control device of the incubator. For mature neonates tested at an environmental temperature of 30.2-32.2°C, temperature at the test site (volar surface of forearm) was similar to that of the premature subjects, as was core temperature and relative humidity. A standard thermal stimulus of 41.5 ± 0.3°C was applied for 10 min. At the end of the heating period sweating was visualized by Wada's method [15]. When positive reactions occurred they were seen within 1-3 min, rarely extending beyond the 15 mm diameter of heating by more than 2-3 mm during the 10 min observation period. Eighteen of 26 full-term infants had positive sweating responses, and only four of 18 premature infants showed positive reactions, $\chi^2 = 5.99$, with one degree of freedom, $P < 0.02$.

For 18 mature infants tested at three lower ambient temperature ranges, 28-29.3°C, 25.8-26.5°C, and 23.8-24.9°C, positive sweating reactions were elicited at each range of ambient temperature. The effect of inhibition of local thermal sweating reactions by a cold environment could not be shown. Distribution of sweating responses are shown for birth weight and gestational age in Figure 8.

Sweat gland responsiveness was also tested with intradermal injection of either adrenaline or acetylcholine 10^{-3} in a 0.02 ml dose. Only one of 44 mature neonates failed to respond to pharmacologic stimulation. Sweating reactions could be elicited in 10 out of 11 mature infants who were unable to produce sweat in response to local heating. For 21 low-birth-weight babies who were predominantly born prior to term, all six who had positive sweating responses to heat had positive reactions to pharmacologic stimulation. Among

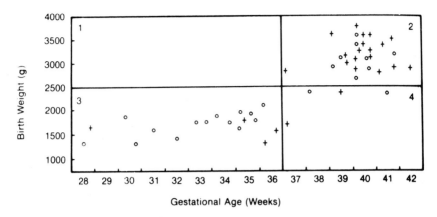

Figure 8 Sweating responses of 48 neonates relative to birth weight and gestational age to a standard thermal stimulus. +, positive reaction; ○, negative reaction. (*Source*: from Green M, Behrendt H: Am J Dis Child, 125:20-25, 1973. Copyright 1973, American Medical Association.)

the 15 who were unresponsive to application of heat, six showed positive responses to sudorific drugs. In no instance was the thermal stimulus effective in infants refractory to stimulation with sudorific drugs. The lack of responsiveness to local heat in the neonate does not necessarily indicate total refractoriness of the end-organ. Moreover, it is not warranted to assume that the greater responsiveness of the sweat gland to local pharmacological stimulation indicates that the neural reflex component evoked by local thermal stimulation is deficient in the term neonate since it is not possible to define the comparative intensity of the different modes of stimulation. Nevertheless, an active neural component was confirmed in the mature newborn. Prior intracutaneous injection of 0.2 ml of 1% procaine caused diminution of the sweating response to local heating. The effect was demonstrated at both low and high environmental temperatures. The lack of inhibition of the sweating response to heat at the lower environmental temperature as found in adults [7] may be due to the fact that neonates were not exposed to temperatures as low as the adults.

That the mature neonate has impairment of sweating in response to local heating has been shown by the results of tests carried out on 10 full-term infants compared with those reported for adults tested at similar environmental temperature and with equivalent intensity of thermal stimulation [36]. None of the infants was able to show sweating reactions to a local heating stimulus of 38.7°C for 10 min; for adults the mean time threshold capable of evoking a positive sweating response was 3 min. For a thermal stimulus of approximately

Table 1 Comparative Time Thresholds for Local Thermal Stimulation of Sweating in Neonates and Adults

	Ambient temperature ($^{\circ}$C)	Relative humidity (%)	Heating temperature ($^{\circ}$C)	Mean time threshold (min)
10 full-size neonates	27.7 (26.8-28.5)	30-50	38.7	10
10 adults[a]	27.8	65	38.3	3.0
10 full-size neonates	27.7 (26.8-28.5)	30-50	41.5	6.1
10 adults[a]	27.8	65	41.4	2.0

[a]From Benjamin

Source: M. Green and H. Behrendt, *Am J Dis Child* 125:20-25, 1973. Copyright 1973, American Medical Association.

41.5°C the mean time threshold was more than 6 min in newborn infants and only 2 min for adults (Table 1).

The ability to produce local sweating in response to stimulation with heat is not fully developed in the infant born at term, and the degree of impairment is even greater in the premature infant. There is substantial evidence that sweat gland reactivity depends on sensitivity of the end-organ itself and on a neural factor arising within the central nervous system. In view of the comparability of local sudorific thresholds for adrenaline and acetylcholine in the adult and the mature neonate, a reasonable explanation for the diminished sweating responsiveness to local thermal stimulation in the mature newborn is delay in maturation of the neural component. In the premature infant function of both the sweat gland and the neural pathways is presumed to be defective.

TESTS OF SUDOMOTOR NERVE FUNCTION

Axon Reflex Sweating

Functional competence of the sudomotor nerves can be evaluated by the sudomotor axon reflex. The reflex is mediated solely by the peripheral ramifications of a single postganglionic sympathetic axon. It can be evoked even in the absence of anatomic integrity of neural connections with the central nervous system [30,37]. The reflex can still be obtained even after fresh section of the postganglionic sudomotor nerve but disappears after the onset of the reaction of degeneration distal to the ganglion. Upon stimulation of the neural receptor

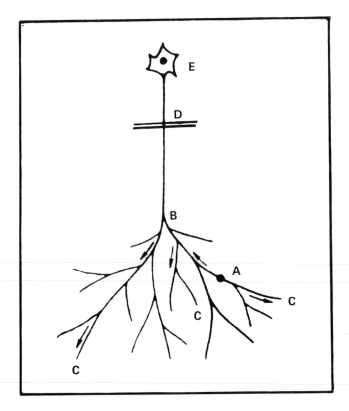

Figure 9 Schema for axon reflex. A, point of reception; B, highest point of ramification; C, nerve endings; D, point of severence; E, ganglion cell. Reflex is not abolished when axon is severed at D by injury or block anesthesia. (*Source*: Ref 39 © 1940, The Williams and Wilkins Company, Baltimore.)

point by intradermal injection of an appropriate pharmacologic agent, impulses first travel centripetally along terminal sudomotor fibers until they reach the highest point of ramification. From this locus the direction of transmission of impulses becomes centrifugal, dispersing over all of the terminal branches to the cholinergic receptors of the innervated glands in the vicinity (Fig. 9). Since the response can be blocked by prior infiltration of the skin with ganglionic blocking agents,* the point of highest ramification may be considered to be functionally equivalent to the sympathetic ganglion [38]. Although it is doubtful that

---

*The sudomotor axon reflex elicited by hypertonic solutions of NaCl is an exception to the inhibitory effect of the ganglionic blocking action of tetraethylammonium [23].

axon reflex sweating occurs physiologically in humans, the ability to induce it by a variety of stimuli may be exploited to assess the integrity of sudomotor nerve function in adults as well as neonates [23,30,37-39]. Included among these are: punctiform faradic stimulation of the skin, acetylcholine and its esters, nicotine, alpha-lobeline, and intradermal hypertonic solutions of NaCl. The sweating response differs from that due to the muscarinic action produced directly on cholinergic receptors of the sweat gland. It is characterized by the sudden appearance of sweating dispersed over a relatively wide area surrounding the often-spared intradermal injection site. Onset occurs within approximately 10-60 sec and reaches its maximum density within 2 min. With acetylcholine, it may be difficult to separate axon reflex sweating due to the nicotinic action of the drug from the gradually evolving response caused by its muscarinic action. Characteristic of the nicotinic effect is the ability of very dilute solutions to evoke the axon reflex response and strong concentrations to inhibit it by a paralyzing action [39]. This reputed inhibitory effect was not confirmed with strong concentrations of acetylcholine by Janowitz and Grossman [38].

Green and Behrendt [40] investigated axon reflex sweating in the neonate to define the competence of sudomotor nerve function at this stage of life. Studies were carried out during the first week of life on 14 full-size infants with a gestational age range of 37-42 weeks and 14 low-birth-weight infants with a gestational age range of 30-37 weeks. Infants were tested in incubators with air temperature continuously adjusted by the servocontrolled thermostat set to maintain temperature on the volar surface of the forearm (test site) between 34 and 35°C. Rectal temperature ranged from 36.2-37°C. Relative humidity for individual tests measured between 40 and 70%. Since it might be difficult to determine the efficacy of the sudomotor axon reflex in anhidrotic premature infants, competence for the axon reflex response to intradermal histamine was also tested. Even though the latter reflex is mediated by sensory nerve fibers [41]; if intact, it would provide an estimate of the efficacy of peripheral neural transmission. Nicotine was used to test the sudomotor axon reflex. Since acetylcholine promotes sweating by a dual action it was not selected for this purpose to prevent misinterpretation of sudorific responses. Dilutions of nicotine ranging from 10^{-4} to 10^{-6} (w/v) were prepared with physiological NaCl. A solution of histamine phosphate 10^{-4} (w/v) was prepared with the same diluent for the purpose of testing the vasodilator axon reflex. Of 14 full-size infants, 12 had positive responses to concentrations of nicotine of 10^{-4} or 10^{-5}; in no instance was there a response to the 10^{-6} dilution. Only two of the premature infants had positive sudomotor axon reflex responses. All mature and premature infants with positive sudomotor axon reflexes showed concomitant positive sweating reactions to direct glandular stimulation with acetylcholine or adrenaline as did the two mature newborn infants who failed to show the sudomotor axon reflex. The difference in the proportion of positive sudomotor axon

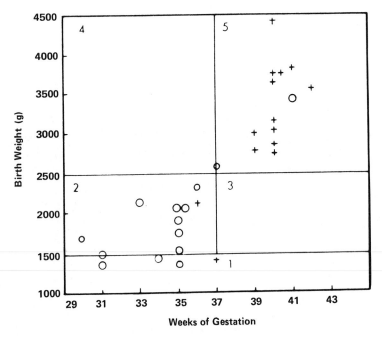

Figure 10 Sweating responses of 28 neonates to nicotine, arranged by birth weight and gestational age groups. +, positive; ○, negative. (*Source*: Green M, Behrendt H: Am J Dis Child 118:725-732, 1969. Copyright 1969, American Medical Association.)

reflexes for each group is highly significant, $\chi^2 = 11.57, P < 0.001$. The distribution of these sweating responses arranged by birth weight and gestation is shown in Figure 10. Eight premature infants who had negative reactions to nicotine showed positive axon reflex flares in response to histamine.

Based on these findings, peripheral sudomotor transmission appears to be intact in the infant born at term and appears to be of a similar order of magnitude to the adult. In contrast, premature infants are unable to demonstrate sudomotor responsiveness just as they fail to show sweating responsiveness to direct stimulation of a refractory end-organ with acetylcholine and adrenaline. Competence of the peripheral sudomotor pathways remains unresolved in infants who appear to be incapable of sweating. However, the functional integrity of peripheral sensory nerve fibers appears to be clearly established even in prematurely born infants by the model of the histamine flare reaction. This finding may not warrant the assumption that sympathetic motor fibers are equivalently competent. Studies eliciting the pilomotor axon reflex may help to resolve this issue.

COMPETENCE OF SWEATING CENTERS

Substantial evidence shows [1-3,9] that generalized sweating in response to environmental thermal stimulation is elicited at a lower temperature range in young adults* whether male or female, than in mature newborns. Experimental studies designed to measure the functional efficiency of the individual components of the sweating apparatus [19,32,35,40] have produced evidence that this neonatal handicap is probably not due exclusively to inefficacy of the sweat gland. It appears more difficult to explain the reason for the anhidrosis of prematurely born infants; since the sweat gland of the immature infant is refractory to stimulation with acetylcholine, the natural neurotransmitter, it is difficult to implicate the operation of additional factors.

The control center for generalized sweating is in the hypothalamus, and although a variety of stimuli can initiate afferent impulse transmission, it is not clear which is the primal one. Temperature of the skin surface, subdermal region, skeletal muscles, and core may all be capable of initiating the afferent limb of the reflex pathway. From the hypothalamic center afferent fibers descend via the brain stem and spinal cord, crossing at various levels and finally terminating in the lateral horns. Preganglionic neurons in this region emerge from the cord to synapse with neurons in the paravertebral sympathetic ganglia. Postganglionic sudomotor fibers originating here pass via the gray rami communicantes to the spinal nerves and terminate at the periglandular junction.

Anomalies of the Central Nervous System

Information on degree of competence of sweating centers in the newborns has been derived from studies of young infants with congenital malformations of the central nervous system. Foster et al. [43] evaluated sweating capacity in 50 infants, 26 of whom were less than 1 month of age and 10 less than 3 months. Local sweating responsiveness to intradermally administered acetylcholine or iontophoresis of pilocarpine was determined by starch-iodine paper prints and by measurement of the increment of water content of the effluent air from a capsule applied to the skin. Conditions such as anencephaly, hydranencephaly, encephalocoele, and hydrocephalus tended to be associated with anhidrosis in

---

*Sweating responsiveness of elderly people to pharmacological stimulation with acetylcholine or methacholine has been reported to be impaired. Moreover, it has been speculated that relative anhidrosis may cause death due to high environmental temperature in this susceptible age range [42].

spite of elevation of air temperature to levels associated with rectal temperature as high as 37.8°C. In healthy mature newborns, the critical level of rectal temperature for generalized sweating produced by heat is 37.5°C [3]. In addition to impaired generalized sweating, local pharmacological stimulation of sweating tended to be inhibited in spite of administration of doses known to be effective in healthy mature newborns [19]. Infants with meningomyelocoele often demonstrated anhidrosis below the level of the lesion both to environmental temperature and pharmacological stimulation of the sweat gland. In four infants with large occipital encephalocoeles, thermoregulation as well as sweating competence was impaired. In one young infant with impaired sweating function caused by extreme hydrocephalus, the pilomotor axon reflex to nicotine was intact, suggesting that anhidrosis was not due to defective peripheral sudomotor transmission.

In contrast to the anhidrosis characteristic of congenital lesions of preganglionic sympathetic pathways, acquired preganglionic lesions of adults are associated with continued responsiveness of sweat glands to local pharmacological stimulation but loss of thermal reflex sweating [44]. This indicates that integrity of neural structures from the central nervous system to the peripheral neuroglandular junction is necessary for normal functional maturation of eccrine sweat glands. Although the relevant anatomic connections exist in the anhidrotic premature infant, their successful activation requires the completion of gestation and perhaps an additional extrauterine interval when thermal stress may augment sweating capacity to the level found in the adult.

The Neonatal Heroin Withdrawal Syndrome

In the neonatal heroin withdrawal syndrome, signs of illness suggest involvement of the central and autonomic nervous system. A high proportion of these infants become ill shortly after the placental supply of heroin has ended at birth. Among these signs are: coarse tremors, shrill crying, hypertonicity, tachypnea, vomiting, diarrhea, sneezing, and hyperpyrexia. Generalized sweating may also be observed, even at environmental temperature below the neutral thermal range of 32-34°C established for healthy neonates [9]. Behrendt and Green [45] were struck by the occurrence of profuse generalized sweating even in prematurely born infants with this syndrome. In one instance they observed sweating so profuse that the outline of the baby's body could be discerned on the underlying mattress cover. Local sweat gland responsiveness to intradermal pharmacologic agents appeared to be a potentially fruitful area of study based on these observations. Subsequently, they determined sweating thresholds for adrenaline, acetylcholine, and nicotine in untreated addicted neonates and compared these with thresholds for healthy newborns. In a preliminary study they tested both groups of babies for background sweating by means of Wada's starch-iodine technique [15] or by sweat prints made with bromphenol-blue-impregnated paper [46]. These observations were made with infants kept in incubators with air temperature set below the thermal threshold for generalized sweating of 35-37°C found for mature newborns [9]. All low-birth-weight infants were maintained at ambient temperature of 31-34°C and full-size infants were maintained at air temperature of 29-31°C. The low-birth-weight infants were, for the most part, born prematurely and the full-size infants were predominantly born at term. Infants were 1-8 days of age. The frequency of generalized sweating is shown in Table 2. Approximately 23% of healthy mature neonates and less than 2% of healthy premature infants showed spontaneous generalized sweating. In contrast, 40% of addicted low-birth-weight premature infants had spontaneous sweating. Only in the addicted neonates was hyperhidrosis visible in the resting state. The difference in the proportion of spontaneously perspiring addicted infants was significantly higher even than that found for mature unaddicted babies, $\chi^2 = 5.991$ with a confidence coefficient greater than 0.95 and two degrees of freedom.

Stimulation of local sweating activity was carried out by the usual threshold method, using adrenaline and acetylcholine for sweat gland stimulation and nicotine for the sudomotor axon reflex in the same 20 addicted premature newborns and in a group of 26 healthy premature controls. All infants were placed in incubators with abdominal skin temperature thermostatically controlled at 36°C. The range of temperature on the test site measured at the end of a 2 hr adaptation period was comparable for both groups of subjects with means of 34.4°C and 34.7°C for healthy and addicted groups, respectively. Tests were considered invalid if background sweating appeared during testing. Only the muscarinic response to acetylcholine was accepted as evidence of a positive reaction to this drug. The presence of sweat was detected by the starch-iodine reaction [15]. Differential responsiveness to these pharmacological agents for the two groups of subjects is summarized in Table 3. Actual thresholds in relation to gestational age are shown in Figure 11. The difference between the proportion of positive reactors for all three drugs is significantly greater in the addicted than the healthy premature infants, $\chi^2 = 7.815$ with a confidence coefficient greater than 0.95 and three degrees of freedom. The sweat glands and sudomotor nerves of addicted premature neonates show an abnormally high degree of reactivity to pharmacological stimulation, and with increasing gestational age thresholds decrease more sharply in these infants than in healthy control infants.

AN EXPLANATION FOR THE NEONATAL SWEATING HANDICAP

The clinical model of the neonatal heroin withdrawal syndrome permits a rational explanation for the relative anhidrosis of mature neonates and the

Table 2 Frequency of Generalized Sweating in Neonates 1-8 Days Old

Series[a]	Range of gestational age (wk)	Range of birth weight (g)	Total tested	No. positive	No. positive total	Difference	Lower confidence limit[b]
A	39-42	>2500	131	30	0.2290		
B	27-39	936-2466	108	2	0.0185	0.211	0.116
C	27-39	907-2390	20	8	0.4000	0.382	0.110

[a] A, healthy full-size; B, healthy low-birth-weight; C, addicted low-birth-weight infants.
[b] Calculated with a confidence coefficient > 0.95 and 2 degrees of freedom ($\chi^2 = 5.991$) for multiple comparisons.

Source: Reprinted, by permission of *The New England Journal of Medicine,* 286: 1376-1379, 1972.

Table 3 Comparison of Sweating Responsiveness to Epinephrine, Acetylcholine, and Nicotine in Addicted and Healthy Neonates 1-8 Days of Age

Series[a]	Range gestational age (wk)	Total tested	No. positive[b]	No. negative[c]	No. positive total	Difference	Lower confidence limit[d]
Epinephrine							
A	30-37	23	7	16	0.304		
C	27-37	18	13	5	0.722	0.418	0.019
Acetylcholine							
A	28-37	26	4	22	0.154		
C	28-37	15	11	4	0.733	0.579	0.205
Nicotine							
A	31-37	15	2	13	0.133		
C	34-37	10	7	3	0.700	0.567	0.094

[a]A, healthy; C, addicted infants.

[b]Showing thresholds of 1.0 mg/ml or less for epinephrine and acetylcholine, 0.1 mg/ml or less for nicotine.

[c]Nonresponsive to strongest concentrations of sudorific drugs used: threshold concentration > 1.0 mg/ml for epinephrine and acetylcholine, > 0.1 mg/ml for nicotine.

[d]Calculated with confidence coefficient > 0.95 ($\chi^2 = 7.815$), and 3 degrees of freedom for multiple comparisons involving hypotheses on 3 drugs.

Source: Reprinted by permission of *The New England Journal of Medicine* 286:1376-1379, 1972.

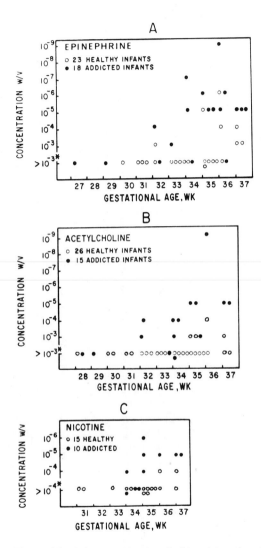

Figure 11 (A) Sweating thresholds with epinephrine in 23 healthy and 18 addicted neonates arranged by gestational age. (B) Sweating thresholds with acetylcholine in 26 healthy and 15 addicted neonates arranged by gestational age. (C) Sweating thresholds with nicotine in 15 healthy and 10 addicted neonates arranged by gestational age. ○, healthy; ●, addicted. (*Source*: Reprinted, by permission of *The New England Journal of Medicine*, 286:1376–1379, 1972.)

tendency towards total anhidrosis in premature infants. The morphologically mature and potentially functional sweat gland will normally remain unresponsive as long as stimulation from immature centers is lacking. However, the sweating defect of prematurity is not immutably fixed. Hyperhidrosis as well as early activation of sweat gland and sudomotor function is provoked by the patho-physiologic disturbances in sudorific centers brought about by the withdrawal syndrome. This is consistent with other signs implicating the central and auto-nomic nervous system in this disorder. The illness causes increased tonicity of sudomotor nerve fibers providing the tonic innervation that according to Roth-man's concept [47], sustains glandular reactivity and renders the end-organ sus-ceptible to direct pharmacological stimulation. There is also generation of actual nerve impulses, presumably from premature activation of centers governing re-flex sweating. It is uncertain whether the generalized hyperhidrosis encountered in these premature infants is exclusively initiated by a lower thermal threshold. It is obviously appropriate to consider this an example of nervous sweating in the neonate. The suggested explanation is not inconsistent with the sweating deficit found with congenital lesions of the central nervous system reported by Foster et al. [43]. Just as an intact central nervous system is a prerequisite for the development of normal sweat gland responsiveness, an intact central nervous system whose activity has been intensified is capable of promoting exaggerated sweat gland reactivity prematurely. A critical duration of gestation may be re-quired before sweat gland activity can be excited. This is reflected by the failure of addicted prematurely born babies of less than 32 weeks of gestation to show sweat gland responsiveness.

COMPOSITION OF ECCRINE SWEAT

Clinical interest in the composition of eccrine sweat was excited by the discovery of the high concentration of sodium chloride in patients with cystic fibrosis [48]. Measurement of sweat sodium and/or chloride has since become the most prac-tical application of knowledge about the composition of eccrine sweat. Volumes of sweat sufficient for measurement can be obtained by pilocarpine iontophore-sis as early as the first day of life in infants born at term [49,50]. Measurements can be made on samples as small as 30 mg [49]. Sweat is collected on preweighed salt-free gauze or filter paper pads placed on the test site and covered with a plastic film to prevent evaporation during the collection period of approximately 30 min. It is then leached with ion-free water and sodium is measured by flame photometry and chloride is determined titrimetrically. Less accurate methods employing ion-specific electrodes and requiring less sweat have been used to take measurements directly from the sweating skin surface of newborns [51].

In healthy neonates, sweat sodium and chloride concentrations are equivalent to those found in normal children [49,50], although both sodium and chloride levels tend to be increased during the first 2 days of life to concentrations as high as 85 mEq/liter and 86 mEq/liter, respectively, [50] before declining to the physiological range of less than 70 mEq/liter for sodium and less than 60 mEq/ liter for chloride [52]. Although elevated levels of potassium have also been observed in neonates with cystic fibrosis [49] and in older children [52], increased concentration is not present as uniformly as is that of sodium and chloride.

The high salt content of eccrine sweat in cystic fibrosis is due to a defect in the duct epithelium. Normally the secretory coil produces an ultrafiltrate of plasma, which undergoes a decrease in concentration in passage through the duct by the combined action of a cellular sodium pump and the passive diffusion of water from the lumen to the periductular tissue [53-55].

Absence of the capacity to sweat poses an obvious obstacle to establishing the time of origin of the defect in the prematurely born infant. This difficulty impedes comparisons for other chemical compounds found in the sweat of adults. Studies on the composition of other products of sweat secretion have not been carried out in the mature newborn.

THE ROLE OF THE ECCRINE SWEAT GLAND IN INSENSIBLE WATER LOSS

In the adult and the mature newborn, insensible water loss takes place from eccrine sweat glands, the extraglandular surface of the epidermis, and the mucosal surface of the respiratory tract. The proportion contributed by the sweat gland is presumed to be nonexistent in the immature newborn incapable of demonstrating visible secretion of sweat. Although the contribution of insensible sweating to total insensible water loss from the skin has been determined in adults by measuring the respective amounts produced before and after atropinization [56], estimation of the proportion of the glandular to the total insensible water loss has not been determined in the mature newborn. It remains to be determined whether the proportion provided by invisible sweating is comparatively less than that for the adult. In the adult the contribution by the sweat gland has been reported to be less in females and in the aged [1,57]. The glandular proportion is also decreased by familiarity of adult subjects with the procedure for measurement of insensible water loss [56]. Because of factors that are likely to cause variability of insensible perspiration in adults, determining the role of the eccrine sweat gland in insensible water loss from the skin of the newborn infant seems a formidable task. For the mature neonate, the capacity for insensible perspiration may reflect the high threshold for visible reflex sweating.

Recently the subject of insensible water loss has become a matter of some concern in the care of newborns, particularly with respect to the survival of prematurely born babies [58-64]. Studies in neonates have been carried out to define the effect of environmental factors on insensible water loss and to determine the contribution of insensible water loss to metabolic rate and total water loss from the body [58,60,64]. Of some importance is the finding that insensible water loss is inversely proportional to gestational age [60,64]. In view of the established anhidrosis of premature infants of less than 34 weeks of gestation, insensible water loss at this stage of life is predominantly if not exclusively derived from sources other than the sweat gland.

REFERENCES

1. Hardy JD, Milhorat AT, DuBois EF: Basal metabolism and heat loss of young women at temperature from 22C to 35C. J Nutrition 21:383-404, 1941.
2. Uchino S: Sweating of newborn infants. Sanka Fujinka Kiyo 22:238-267, 1939.
3. Foster KG, Hey EN, Katz G: The response of the sweat glands of the newborn baby to thermal stimuli and intradermal acetylcholine. J Physiol 203: 13-29, 1969.
4. Szabo G: The number of eccrine sweat glands in human skin. Adv Biol Skin 3:1-5, 1962.
5. Kawahata A: Numerical studies on the human active sweat glands. Nippon Seirigaku-Zasshi 4:438, 1939.
6. Borsetto PL: Osservazioni sullo sviluppo delle ghiandole sudoripare nelle diverse regioni della cute umana. Arch Ital Anat Embriol 56:332-348, 1951.
7. Issekutz Jr B, Hetenyi Jr G, Diosy A: Contributions to the physiology of sweat secretion. Arch Int Pharmacodyn 83:133-142, 1950.
8. Randall WC: Local sweat gland activity to direct effects of radiant heat. Am J Physiol 150:365-371, 1947.
9. Bruck K: Temperature regulation in the newborn infant. Biol Neonate 3: 65-119, 1961.
10. McLaughlin JT, Sonnenschein RR: Response of human sweat glands to local heating. J Invest Dermatol 41:27-29, 1963.
11. von Beaumont W, Bullard RW: Direct influence of temperature. Science 147:1465-1467, 1965.
12. Janowitz HD, Grossman MI: The response of the sweat glands to some locally acting agents in human subjects. J Invest Dermatol 14:453-458, 1950.
13. Randall WC, Kimura KK: Pharmacology of sweating. Pharmacol Rev 7: 365-397, 1955.
14. Haimovici H: Evidence for an adrenergic component in the nervous mechanism of sweating in man. Proc Soc Exp Biol Med 68:40-41, 1948.

15. Wada M: Sudorific action of adrenalin on the human sweat glands and determination of their excitability. Science 111:376-377, 1950.

16. Chalmers TM, Keele CA: Physiological significance of the sweat response to adrenaline in man. J Physiol 114:510-514, 1951.

17. Sonnenschein RR, Kobrin H, Janowitz HD, Grossman MI: Stimulation and inhibition of human sweat glands by intradermal sympathomimetic agents. J. Appl Physiol. 3:573-581, 1951.

18. Hurley HJ, Wittkowski JA: Mechanism of epinephrine-induced eccrine sweating in human skin. J Appl Physiol 16:652-654, 1961.

19. Behrendt H, Green M: Drug-induced localized sweating in full-size and low-birth-weight neonates. Am J Dis Child 117:299-306, 1969.

20. Wada M, Takagaki T: A simple and accurate method for detecting the secretion of sweat. Tohoku J Exp Med 49:284, 1948.

21. Haimovici H: Evidence for adrenergic sweating in man. J Appl Physiol 2:512-521, 1950.

22. Sonnenschein RR, Kobrin H, Grossman MI: Further observations on local action of epinephrine on human sweat glands. Am J Physiol 159:591-592, 1949.

23. Wada M, Arai T, Takagaki T, Nakagawa T: Axon reflex mechanism in sweat responses to nicotine, acetylcholine, and sodium chloride. J Appl Physiol 4:745-752, 1952.

24. Behrendt H, Green M: Unpublished observations, 1973.

25. Gibson LE: Personal communication with H Behrendt, 1974.

26. Gibson LE: The effect of adrenergic stimulation upon sweating in normal children and cystic fibrosis patients. Pediatrics 42:458-464, 1968.

27. Beckett EB, Bourne GH, Montagna W: Histology and cytochemistry of human skin. The distribution of cholinesterase in the finger of the embryo and the adult. J Physiol 134:202-206, 1956.

28. Uno H, Montagna W: Catecholamine-containing nerve terminals of the eccrine sweat glands of Macaques. Cell Tissue Res 158:1-13, 1975.

29. Foster KG, Weiner JS: Effects of cholinergic and adrenergic blocking agents on the activity of the eccrine sweat glands. J Physiol 210:883-895, 1970.

30. Coon JM, Rothman S: The sweat response to drugs with nicotine-like action. J Pharmacol Exp Ther 73:1-11, 1941.

31. Collins KJ, Sargent F, Weiner JS: Excitation and depression of eccrine sweat glands by acetylcholine, acetyl-B-methyl-choline, and adrenalin. J Physiol 148:592-614, 1959.

32. Green M, Behrendt H: Drug-induced sweating in neonates. Responses to exogenous and endogenous acetylcholine. Am J Dis Child 120:434-438, 1970.

33. Green M, Behrendt H: Sweat gland reactivity to local thermal stimulation in dysautonomia. Am J Dis Child 130:816-818, 1976.

34. Riley CM: Familial dysautonomia. Adv Pediatr 9:157-190, 1957.

35. Green M, Behrendt H: Sweating responses of neonates to local thermal stimulation. Am J Dis Child 125:20-25, 1973.
36. Benjamin FB: Sweating response to local heat application. J Appl Physiol 5:594-598, 1953.
37. Sonnenschein RR, Bernstein M: Relation to the central nervous system of neural pathways mediating histamine flare and nicotine sweating. J Appl Physiol 11:481-485, 1957.
38. Janowitz H, Grossman MI: Blocking action of tetraethyl-ammonium on axon reflexes in the human skin. Science 109:16, 1949.
39. Rothman S, Coon JM: Axon reflex responses to acetylcholine in the skin. J Invest Dermatol 3:79-97, 1940.
40. Green M, Behrendt H: Sweating capacity of neonates. Nicotine-induced axon reflex sweating and the histamine flare. Am J Dis Child 118:725-732, 1969.
41. Lewis T: *The Blood Vessels of the Human Skin and Their Responses.* Shaw, London, 1927, pp 59-71.
42. Ellis FP, Exton-Smith AN, Foster KG, Weiner JS: Eccrine sweating and mortality during heat waves in very young and very old persons. Israel J Med Sci 12:815-817, 1976.
43. Foster KG, Hey EN, O'Connell B: Sweat function in babies with defects of the central nervous system. Arch Dis Child 46:444-451, 1971.
44. Chalmers TM, Keele CA: The nervous and chemical control of sweating. Br J Dermatol 64:43-54, 1952.
45. Behrendt H, Green M: Nature of the sweating defect of prematurely born neonates. Observations on babies with the heroin withdrawal syndrome. N Engl J Med 286:1376-1379, 1972.
46. Sakurai M, Montagna W: The skin of primates XVII. Pharmacological properties of the sweat gland of Lemur mongoz. J Invest Dermatol 42:411-414, 1964.
47. Rothman S: *Physiology and Biochemistry of the Skin.* University of Chicago Press, Chicago, 1954, p 165.
48. di Sant'Agnese PA, Darling RC, Perera GA, Shea E: Abnormal electrolyte composition of sweat in cystic fibrosis of the pancreas; clinical significance and relationship to disease. Pediatrics 12:549-563, 1953.
49. Elian E, Schwachman H, Hendren WH: Intestinal obstruction of the newborn infant. Usefulness of the sweat electrolyte test in differential diagnosis. N Engl J Med 264:13-15, 1961.
50. Stur O: Electrolyte concentrations in the sweat of the newborn. Neue Oest Z Kinderheilk 6:347-355, 1961.
51. Warwick W: Cystic fibrosis sweat test for newborns. JAMA 198:59-62, 1966.
52. di Sant'Agnese PA, Gibson LE: The eccrine sweat defect in cystic fibrosis of the pancreas. Adv Biol Skin 3:229-255, 1962.

53. Schulz IJ: Micropuncture studies of sweat formation in cystic fibrosis patients. J Clin Invest 48:1470-1477, 1969.
54. Sato K: Sweat induction from an isolated eccrine sweat gland. Am J Physiol 225:1147-1151, 1973.
55. Brusilow SW, Gordes EH: Determination of sweat gland precursor fluid osmolarity by direct cryoscopy. J Clin Invest 42:920-921, 1963.
56. Rothman S: *Physiology and Biochemistry of the Skin.* University of Chicago Press, Chicago, 1965, p 236.
57. Jores A: Perspiratio insensibilis, III. Z Gesamte Exp Med 77:734-742, 1931.
58. Hey EN, Katz G: Evaporative water loss in the newborn baby. J Physiol 200:605-619, 1969.
59. Oh W, Karecki H: Phototherapy and insensible water loss in the newborn infant. Am J Dis Child 124:230-232, 1972.
60. Fanaroff AA, Wald M, Gruber HS, Klauss MH: Insensible water loss in low birth weight infants. Pediatrics 50:236-245, 1972.
61. Wu PYK, Hodgman JE: Insensible water loss in preterm infants. Changes with postnatal development and non-ionizing radiant energy. Pediatrics 54:704-712, 1974.
62. Williams PR, Oh W: Effect of radiant warmer on insensible water loss in newborn infants. Am J Dis Child 128:511-514, 1974.
63. Oh W: Disorders of fluids and electrolytes in newborn infants. Pediatr Clin North Am 23:601-609, 1976.
64. Marks KH, Friedman Z, Maisels MJ: A simple device for reducing insensible water loss in low-birth-weight infants. Pediatrics 60:223-226, 1977.

3

The Sebaceous Gland

PETER E. POCHI
Boston University Medical Center, Boston, Massachusetts

The sebaceous glands occur in the skin of all mammalian species [1]. Their function is to provide a mantle of lipid (sebum) to coat the fur as a protection against overwetting and for heat insulation. Also, in many species, specialized sebaceous structures have evolved, the secretions of which contain pheromones for territorial marking and sexual attraction [2]. In humans, however, these functions of sebum, which provide essential protective properties in other animals, appear to have limited importance insofar as the basic integrity of the skin is concerned [3].

DEVELOPMENT

Morphologically, the sebaceous gland is a multiacinar, holocrine-secreting tissue found in all areas of the skin, except for the palms, soles, and dorsum of the feet [4]. The glands are associated with hair follicles from which they derive embryologically and form the pilosebaceous unit structure in the skin. Human sebaceous glands first form in the skin in the 4th month of gestation as budding cells from the follicular primordium [5,6]. Full maturation of organelles in the sebaceous gland cells occurs by the 6th month, ultrastructural study showing features essentially similar to those of the adult [6]. However, it is not known whether glandular *size,* and thereby secretory capacity, continues to increase further until birth. In any event, the sebaceous secretion contributes a significant proportion of the vernix caseosa, the variably adherent fetal skin-surface

Table 1 Skin Surface Lipid Levels at Various Ages

Subjects		Casual level (forehead) (mg/10 cm^2)
Neonates	20	1.67 (0.92-2.10)
Children	15	0.46 (0.00-0.98)
Men	20	1.24 (0.93-1.78)
Women	20	0.94 (0.63-1.38)

Source: Data from Ref. 14.

film consisting of lipids, epidermal cells, water, and other substances from the amniotic fluid [7]. Desquamating sebaceous gland cells are found in amniotic fluid and can be detected by their orange-pink to brown cytoplasmic stain with Nile blue sulfate, in contrast to the light blue appearance of shed epidermal cells with the same stain [8]. The finding of sebaceous gland cells with intact nuclei in the amniotic fluid is of interest, since in the skin one sees characteristically on histologic examination that mature lipid-laden sebaceous gland cells become anucleate and disrupt, with disgorgement of their sebum prior to their excretion into the follicular canal [4,9].

In contrast to the many studies of the sebaceous glands and their secretory activity in adolescents and adults [4,10-12], studies of children, and particularly of infants in the neonatal period, have been few. At birth, the sebaceous glands are large although not as voluminous or multilobulated as in the adult [13]. Emanuel [14] examined surface lipid levels in the newborn and found casual levels to be comparatively high at birth in contrast to those of children (Table 1) In fact, they were even higher than those of adults. To obviate the problem of contaminant vernix caseosa adding to the true sebum level, samples were taken at 8 days as well as at 24-48 h after birth, and similar results were obtained. However, the possible additive effect from vernix caseosa cannot be absolutely excluded, as it may adhere to some extent on the skin for longer than a week [7]. Agache et al. [15] have also found casual surface lipid levels to be higher at birth. They further determined them to be greater in male than in female infants, supporting an earlier reported observation that sebum lipids in vernix caseosa show a similar male preponderance [16].

By measuring the relative composition of skin surface lipids [17], it is possible to confirm that the high quantity of perinatal surface lipids is due to sebaceous gland secretion. Skin surface lipid derives from two principal sources: sebum and epidermal lipid. It is a complex mixture of triglycerides, mono- and diglycerides, fatty acids, wax esters, squalene, sterols, sterol esters, and diol esters [18]. The composition of sebum and of epidermal lipid is different, with

Table 2 Skin Surface Lipid Composition (%) (Forehead)

Age	Wax esters (WE)	Sterols+sterol esters (S+SE)	WE/(S+SE)	Free fatty acids
5 d	26.7	8.6	3.10	1.5
1 mo–2 yr	17.6	14.0	1.26	20.8
2–4 yr	8.0	13.1	0.61	22.9
4–8 yr	6.9	21.8	0.32	15.9
8–10 yr	17.8	8.9	2.00	17.8
10–15 yr	23.6	6.0	3.93	18.8
18–40 yr	25.0	3.5	7.14	16.4

Source: Ref. 20. © The Williams & Wilkins Co., Baltimore.

wax esters and squalene synthesized only by the sebaceous gland. Sterols and sterol esters are primarily products of epidermal keratinization. Glycerides are found in both tissues. In sebaceous-rich areas, such as the face, approximately 95% of the surface lipid film is sebum with the small remainder being epidermal lipid [19]. Here, maximum amounts of wax esters will be found with correspondingly low values for sterols and sterol esters. When the contribution of sebum is small, these percentages tend to reverse. In eight newborns, from whom forehead surface lipid was collected at day 5 following daily hexachlorophene cleansing from birth, it could be shown that the percentage of wax esters was comparable to that of the adult [20] (Table 2). The same trend for an adult simulated composition was seen for percentages of sterols plus sterol esters and for the ratio of wax esters to them, although the percentages of epidermal lipid contribution appeared higher at birth than in the adult, again possibly due to a small amount of persisting vernix. Table 2 also shows a very low percentage of free fatty acids in the early surface lipid film, probably a reflection of negligible microbial growth at this stage of life. Studies of isolated sebaceous glands [21] and of regional differences in surface lipid composition [19] indicate that free fatty acids are absent in newly secreted sebum but are formed from intrafollicular glyceride lipolysis, presumably as a result of microbial lipase action.

After birth, glandular size and secretion decrease. By measuring the fatty acid ester content of the forehead of newborns, 3-month-old, and 12-month-old infants, Blecha et al. [22] found lipid levels to decrease progressively at 3 and 12 months of age (Table 3). Cross-sectional studies [15], in which casual surface lipid samples have been examined in a large number of newborns and infants, show that the comparatively high levels at birth fall by the 2nd and 3rd month and appear to stabilize at approximately 6 months of age. However, Table 2

Table 3 Esterified Fatty Acid Content
($\mu g/cm^2$) of Skin Surface Lipid

Age	N	Forehead	Chest
Newborn	11	718.0	167.1
3 mo	10	146.5	85.9
12 mo	10	89.0	53.1

Source: Data from Ref. 22.

Table 4 Wax Esters/(Sterols + Sterol Esters) Ratio in Skin Surface Lipid
(Forehead) Mean ± SD (Coefficient of Variation)

Age (yr)	Males	Females
5	0.25 ± 0.09 (36.0%)	0.24 ± 0.03 (12.5%)
6	0.24 ± 0.13 (54.1%)	1.13 ± 0.95 (84.1%)
7	0.92 ± 1.01 (109.8%)	1.43 ± 1.19 (83.2%)
8	1.50 ± 1.26 (84.0%)	2.34 ± 1.69 (72.2%)
9	2.71 ± 1.95 (72.0%)	3.38 ± 2.12 (62.7%)
10	3.86 ± 1.99 (51.6%)	4.37 ± 1.65 (37.8%)
11	5.98 ± 1.89 (31.6%)	5.36 ± 1.80 (33.6%)
12	9.64 ± 2.95 (30.6%)	7.86 ± 2.34 (29.8%)
13	—	8.23 ± 2.48 (30.1%)

shows data to indicate, on the basis of the more sensitive measure of lipid composition, that sebaceous secretion (wax ester content) decreases to reach an essentially stable level not until the second year or so of life. In early childhood,
the sebaceous glands are small [4,23-25], producing small amounts of sebum
[14,20,25-27]; occasionally, a pilosebaceous unit will display an unusually large
gland [24]. The recrudescence of sebaceous gland activity occurs in midchild-
hood. Table 4 shows combined longitudinal and cross-sectional data of the
measurement of forehead sebum, expressed as the wax esters/(sterol+sterol
esters) ratio, in 52 children studied longitudinally for 4 years. At entry into the
study, the subjects ranged in age from 5 to 9 years. Lipid samples were obtained
four times yearly and an average of two consecutive collections assigned a single
value, giving 8 data points (two per year) for each individual. It is evident that
an increase in wax esters occurs at the chronological age of 6 in girls and 7 in
boys. Further rise in secretion takes place with time into early puberty at which

point the activity, as expressed by the ratio, is similar to that of the 18-40 year group of subjects (Table 2). In actuality, however, when measured by 3-hr sebum collection and direct gravimetric assay, sebaceous gland activity can be shown to continue to increase further until the late teens [28].

HORMONAL CONTROL

The development and secretory activity of the sebaceous gland in humans are influenced profoundly by hormonal factors [10,11]. Androgenic steroids are chiefly responsible for this effect, particularly those of testicular or ovarian origin, although adrenal androgens are probably responsible for early sebaceous gland maturation in mid- to late childhood [27]. Glucocorticoids appear to have a permissive role, as may anterior pituitary hormones, although the primary effect of the latter is to influence the sebaceous gland indirectly through stimulation of appropriate target organs, the adrenal cortex, ovaries, and testis [11]. The thyroid gland may be an additional regulator of sebaceous gland activity, since patients with decreased thyroid gland activity show corresponding decreased sebaceous lipid synthesis [29].

The fetal development of the sebaceous gland, observed to occur in the 4th month [5,6] is probably the result of androgenic stimulation. The fetal adrenal cortex develops in the first trimester of pregnancy, with Δ^5-3β-hydroxysteroids predominating because of a relative deficiency of Δ^5-3β-hydroxysteroid dehydrogenase activity [30]. Consequently, large amounts of dehydroepiandrosterone and dehydroepiandrosterone sulfate are formed; these steroids are capable of stimulating sebaceous gland activity [31,32]. Fetal gonadal steroid secretion may also be a factor in the stimulation of the sebaceous gland. Leydig cells first appear in the fetal testis at 8 weeks of age, reaching maximal development at 12-15 weeks [33]. The in vitro synthesis of testosterone by fetal testicular tissue increases between the 9th and 15th week [34]. By comparison, steroid synthetic capacity in fetal ovaries is limited [34,35]. The sexual disparity in androgen biosynthesis is evident at birth; the concentration of testosterone in the cord blood of males is higher than that of females (53.0 and 39.0 ng/dl, respectively [36]). The same relationship holds for the peripheral blood (68.1 and 12.0 ng/dl, respectively). These levels of testosterone are considerably higher than those found in children, the latter of which show mean values of only 6.62 in boys and 6.58 ng/dl in girls [36]. In the first year of life, the concentrations of plasma testosterone show a differential progression as to sex [37]. In male infants, the plasma concentration of testosterone actually increases in the neonatal period whereas that of females shows a decrease (Table 5). After the 3rd month, levels in male infants begin to decline, and by the end of the first year both sexes show the same low levels of testosterone. The unusually

Table 5 Plasma Testosterone Levels (ng/dl) from
Birth to 12 Months of Age

Age	Males	Females
1-15 d	68.1	12.0
1-3 mo	201.6	8.5
3-5 mo	87.5	6.7
5-7 mo	21.5	6.5
7-12 mo	7.6	6.2

Source: Ref. 37.

high levels of circulating testosterone in male infants are not virilizing, presumably because of concomitant increased binding by testosterone estradiol-binding globulin [38].

SURFACE LIPID FILM

The composition of skin surface lipids in the neonate, as mentioned above, shows a pattern similar to that of the adult; a high percentage of wax esters and squalene, lipids of sebaceous gland origin, and a low percentage of epidermal lipids [20]. Detailed studies of the chemistry of the surface lipid film at birth have been limited to examinations of the vernix caseosa; the results of these investigations have been reviewed by Downing and Strauss [18]. The class composition of the lipids in vernix, as published by Kärkkäinen et al. [39], is compared in Table 6 with that of adult skin surface lipid as reported by Ramasastry et al. [20]. The findings in vernix caseosa indicate the presence of sebum, but with a high proportion of epidermal lipid. One might have assumed that this would be the case because of the physical nature of vernix, with its relatively high proportion of cornified cells. However, the findings cannot be totally explained on the basis of a disproportionate amount of epidermal lipid since in vernix caseosa (1) the concentration of total glycerides (glycerides plus free fatty acids) is less than one-half that found in either sebum or epidermal lipid; (2) the ratio of squalene to wax esters exceeds that in sebum; and (3) the ratio of sterol esters/sterols is greater than in epidermal lipid [18]. Additional observations reveal that vernix lipids differ in several other respects from adult skin surface lipid [39-41], namely (1) a higher proportion of branched-chain saturated fatty acids (78% versus 12%); (2) a lower proportion of Δ^6 monounsaturated acids esterified with sterols (30% versus 89%); and (3) a higher proportion of Δ^9 monounsaturated acids esterified with sterols (70% versus 11%) and waxes (12% versus 1%). The chemical compo-

Table 6 Lipid Composition (%) of Vernix Caseosa; Comparison with Adult Surface Lipid

	Vernix caseosa[a]	Adult[b]
Squalene	9.0	12.0
Wax esters	11.7	25.0
Sterols	9.0	1.4
Sterol esters	33.0	2.1
Triglycerides	25.7	57.4
Diol esters	7.3	—
Other	4.3	—

[a]Data from Ref. 39.
[b]Data from Ref. 20.

sition of postnatal sebum is not known, nor when the change to that of the "adult" from the vernix pattern takes place. Whether these differences render one or the other type of lipid more or less protective to the skin is also not known.

PROTECTIVE ROLE OF SEBUM

Sebum's role in providing a physiological function in human skin has not been successfully documented. Kligman has reviewed the work of others and reported his own studies which appear to refute long-held beliefs concerning beneficial properties of sebum, such as its having a barrier function, a moisturizing action via emulsification, an antifungal action, and an antibacterial action [3]. However, Aly et al. have described studies showing evidence of an in vivo antimicrobial action of skin surface lipids (acetone extracts of forearm skin), specifically against *Staphylococcus aureus*, *Streptococcus pyogenes*, and *Candida albicans* [42,43]. To what degree a protective effect is exerted endogenously in response to naturally occurring infections or which lipids account for this phenomenon has not been established. In vitro studies have demonstrated inhibition of *Propionibacterium acnes* by naturally occurring sebaceous lipids, specifically various saturated fatty acids [44] and unsaturated fatty acids [45]. Of interest is the report of Parran and Brinkman demonstrating the in vitro reduction of the antibacterial activity of a variety of antimicrobial substances by a simulated sebum substrate, an action that was usually augmented when free fatty acids were present [46]. Finally, skin surface lipids have been found in vitro to have an insect repellent effect, specifically against the female *Aedes aegypti* mosquito

[47]. The effect resided mostly in the fatty acid fraction, of which the most active insect repellent activity occurred in saturated acids with chain-lengths of less than 13 carbon atoms and in a wide range of unsaturated acids [48]. Interestingly, the most potent fatty acid isolated was 9,12,15-octadecatrienoic acid which Ko et al. [45] found to be the most active inhibitor of the growth of propionibacteria.

The role of sebum in the neonate is even more uncertain. It has long been argued that the vernix caseosa might be protective, but practices have varied as to the appropriateness of its early versus late mechanical removal from the skin. Pediatric texts, including those in the areas of perinatal and neonatal care give scant, and usually oblique or vague, comments concerning the potentially helpful (or harmful) effects of the residual postnatal vernix. What little attention is paid to this matter centers around its possible benefit in preventing infection. Beare and Rook [49] state that "its [vernix caseosa] routine removal is likely to increase the susceptibility to skin infections" but cite no supporting references. The postnatal secretion of sebum remains at a relatively high rate, certainly for the duration of the neonatal period. Should sebum have an as yet unidentified beneficial function, the young infant would continue to bear this protective shield for several weeks of life at the very least.

ALTERATIONS IN DISEASE

Further insight into the role of the sebaceous gland might be gained by its study in various disease states of the skin to observe possible alterations in its activity and/or in the composition of sebum.

Atopic Dermatitis

In atopic dermatitis the dryness of the skin is often attributed anecdotally to reduced sebaceous gland activity. For example, Prose published two strikingly contrasting photos of the differences in the histological appearance of the sebaceous glands between atopic and normal glands [50]. The affected glands were illustrated as being small and showing little lipid differentiation. Rajka [51] studied 3-hr surface lipid production rates from the back of the hands of adults and found significantly lower rates of lipid production in patients with atopic dermatitis (Table 7). At the normally low lipid levels of the region tested, the quantity of lipid is approximately divided equally as to its source of origin between sebum and epidermal lipid [19]. Thus, if the lowered values in atopic dermatitis are truly less than normal (at low rates of sebum, the technical error of the collection procedure is considerable) they may be due to a reduction in epidermal rather than sebaceous lipid synthesis. It had been noted previously that total lipid content in isolated epidermal tissue from the skin of patients

Table 7 Sebum Production (mg/10cm^2/3 hr) Dorsa of Hands

	Age 17 to 39		Age 40 to 65	
	Men	Women	Men	Women
Normal	0.38	0.31	0.25	0.21
Atopic dermatitis	0.17[a]	0.15[b]	—	—
Contact dermatitis	0.24[c]	0.22	0.17	0.12

[a]$P < 0.05$.
[b]$P < 0.001$.
[c]$P < 0.01$.
Source: Ref. 51.

with atopic dermatitis was lower than that of the skin in normal subjects [52]. Moreover, surface lipid levels, measured in the forehead area where approximately 95% of the surface lipid is of sebaceous gland origin [19], were reported to be no different in individuals with atopic dermatitis when compared to normal subjects [53].

Contact Dermatitis

In contact dermatitis, lipid production rates were also lower than normal but significantly different statistically only for men and not for women [51]. By contrast, Gloor et al. determined that surface lipid levels, both by the casual and replacement sum methods of measurement, were not abnormal in patients with contact dermatitis [54]. Vallecchi et al., reported from lipid composition studies that the free fatty acid and squalene content of the surface lipid in patients with contact dermatitis was somewhat lower than normal, 38% and 26% less, respectively [55]. The significance of these observations remains obscure.

Acne Vulgaris

The finding of acne vulgaris at birth or its development in the neonatal period is uncommon but by no means rare and presumably depends on the comparatively high levels of sebum found in the perinatal and neonatal periods (see above). The largest single reported series of infantile acne is that of Bessone who described in detail 43 cases observed in a 15-year period [56]. Several features characterize acne at this stage, namely a male predominance (5:1), localization to the face, especially the cheeks, the rarity of nodular lesions, and the infrequency of scarring, although it can occur. While most cases gradually subside within a few months or up to a year or so, some show continued activity. Some

Table 8 Forehead Surface Lipid Composition (%) in Seven Cases of Infantile Acne

Onset of acne	Age tested (mo)	Sex	Free fatty acids	Triglycerides	Wax esters	Sterols	Sterol esters	Squalene
At birth	3	F	0.2	51.1	24.0	2.7	7.4	14.5
At birth	4	M	24.0	25.1	20.9	3.0	9.3	17.7
3 mo	9	M	10.2	42.3	20.3	1.2	4.9	20.2
4 wk	9	F	0.4	41.2	5.9	7.7	40.9	3.8
At birth	10	M	8.3	65.2	11.7	4.1	4.7	6.0
4 mo	13	M	6.6	54.7	23.4	2.4	6.6	6.2
2 wk	14	M	10.4	48.3	7.6	3.1	14.0	16.0
Mean	9	–	8.6	46.8	16.3	3.5	12.5	12.1
Normal subjects (7)	10	–	20.8	38.4	17.6	3.7	10.3	9.4

cases are due to or aggravated by the application of emollients or, rarely, a consequence of an underlying endocrine disorder. There is no adequate explanation for the development of such miniaturized acne by some infants; it is stated, but without documentation, that such individuals are prone to develop severe juvenile acne subsequently. This might suggest a state of seborrhea in infants with acne. However, studies of lipid composition of the sebum from the forehead of seven infants with acne have shown no significant differences as compared to a group of normal infants, except for an unexplained decreased concentration of free fatty acids (Table 8). Thus, the pathogenetic mechanisms of infantile acne remain unknown and deserve further study.

ACKNOWLEDGMENT

This study was supported in part by U.S. Public Health Service grants AM 07388 and HD 11632.

REFERENCES

1. Montagna W: Comparative aspects of sebaceous glands, in *Advances in Biology of Skin, Vol IV, The Sebaceous Glands*, edited by Montagna W, Ellis RA, and Silver AF. Pergamon Press, Oxford, 1963.
2. Mykytowycz R, Goodrich BS: Skin glands as organs of communication in mammals. J Invest Dermatol 62:124-131, 1974.
3. Kligman AM: The uses of sebum? in *Advances in Biology of Skin, Vol IV, The Sebaceous Glands*, edited by Montagna W, Ellis RA, and Silver AF. Pergamon Press, Oxford, 1963.
4. Strauss JS, Pochi PE: Histology, histochemistry and electron microscopy of sebaceous glands in man. Normale und pathologische Anatomie der Haut I, in *Jadassohn Handb Haut Geschlechtskr Bd I/1*, edited by Gans O and Steigleder GK. Springer-Verlag, Berlin, 1968, pp 184-223.
5. Serri F, Huber WM: The development of sebaceous glands in man, in *Advances in Biology of Skin, Vol IV, The Sebaceous Glands*, edited by Montagna W, Ellis RA, and Silver AF. Pergamon Press, Oxford, 1963.
6. Breathnach AS: *An Atlas of the Ultrastructure of Human Skin. Development, Differentiation and Post-natal Features.* J & A Churchill, London, 1971, pp 335-352.
7. Solomon LM, Esterly NB: Neonatal dermatology, in *Major Problems in Clinical Pediatrics, Vol IX*, edited by Schaffer AJ. Saunders, Philadelphia, 1973.
8. Sharp F: Estimation of fetal maturity by amniotic fluid exfoliative cytology. J Obstet Gynaecol Br Commonw 75:812-815, 1968.

9. Montagna W: The sebaceous glands in man, in *Advances in Biology of Skin, Vol IV, The Sebaceous Glands,* edited by Montagna W, Ellis RA, and Silver AF. Pergamon Press, Oxford, 1963.

10. Shuster S, Thody AJ: The control and measurement of sebum secretion. J Invest Dermatol 62:172-190, 1974.

11. Pochi PE, Strauss JS: Endocrinologic control of the development and activity of the human sebaceous gland. J Invest Dermatol 62:191-201, 1974.

12. Cunliffe WJ, Cotterill JA: *The Acnes. Clinical Features, Pathogenesis and Treatment.* Saunders, London, 1975.

13. Strauss JS, Pochi PE: The hormonal control of human sebaceous glands, in *Advances in Biology of Skin, Vol IV, The Sebaceous Glands,* edited by Montagna W, Ellis RA, and Silver AF. Pergamon Press, Oxford, 1963.

14. Emanuel S: Quantitative determinations of the sebaceous glands' function, with particular mention of the method employed. Acta Dermatol Venereol 17:444-456, 1936.

15. Agache P, Blanc D, Barrand C, Laurent R: Sebum levels during the first year of life. Br J Dermatol 103:643-649, 1980.

16. Nazzaro-Porro M, Passi S, Boniforti L, Belsito F: Effects of aging on fatty acids in skin surface lipids. J Invest Dermatol 73:112-117, 1979.

17. Downing DT: Photodensitometry in the thin-layer chromatographic analysis of neutral lipids. J Chromatogr 38:91-99, 1968.

18. Downing DT, Strauss JS: Synthesis and composition of surface lipids of human skin. J Invest Dermatol 62:228-244, 1974.

19. Downing DT, Greene RS: Double bond positions in the unsaturated fatty acids of vernix caseosa. J Invest Dermatol 50:380-386, 1968.

20. Ramasastry P, Downing DT, Pochi PE, Strauss JS: Chemical composition of human surface lipids from birth to puberty. J Invest Dermatol 54:139-144, 1970.

21. Kellum RE: Human sebaceous gland lipids. Arch Dermatol 59:218-220, 1967.

22. Blecha J, Pazderka J, Frank M: Esterified fatty acids of the skin surface during the first year of life. Cesk Pediatr 18:97-103, 1963.

23. Strauss JS, Pochi PE: The human sebaceous gland: Its regulation by steroidal hormones and its use as an end organ for assaying androgenicity in vivo. Recent Prog Horm Res 19:385-444, 1963.

24. Steigleder GK, Herminghaus O: Zur Struktur der Haut im Kindesalter, im besonderen der Talgdrüsen und der Haare. Arch Klin Exp Dermatol 235:277-283, 1969.

25. Kvorning SA: Investigations into the pharmacology of the skin fats and of ointments. II. On the occurrence and replenishment of fat on the skin in normal individuals. Acta Pharmacol Toxicol 5:262-269, 1949.

26. Pochi PE, Strauss JS, Mescon H: Sebum secretion and urinary fractional 17-ketosteroid and total 17-hydroxycorticoid excretion in male castrates. J Invest Dermatol 39:475-483, 1962.

27. Pochi PE, Strauss JS, Downing DT: Skin surface lipid composition, acne, pubertal development, and urinary excretion of testosterone and 17-keto-steroids in children. J Invest Dermatol 69:485-489, 1977.

28. Pochi PE, Strauss JS, Downing DT: Age-related changes in sebaceous gland activity. J Invest Dermatol 73:108-111, 1979.

29. Goolamali SK, Evered D, Shuster S: Thyroid disease and sebaceous function. Br Med J 1:432-433, 1976.

30. Villee DB: The development of steroidogenesis. Am J Med 53:533-544, 1972.

31. Pochi, PE, Strauss JS: Sebaceous gland response in man to the administration of testosterone, Δ^4-androstenedione, and dehydroisoandrosterone. J Invest Dermatol 52:32-36, 1969.

32. Drucker WD, Blumberg JM, Gandy HM, David RR, Verde AL: Biologic activity of dehydroepiandrosterone sulfate in man. J Clin Endocrinol Metab 35:48-54, 1972.

33. Villee DB: Development of endocrine function in the human placenta and fetus. N Engl J Med 281:533-541, 1969.

34. Bloch E: Metabolism of 4-^{14}C-progesterone by human fetal testis and ovaries. Endocrinology 74:833-845, 1964.

35. Jungmann RA, Schweppe JS: Biosynthesis of sterols and steroids from acetate-^{14}C by human fetal ovaries. J Clin Endocrinol Metab 28:1599-1604, 1968.

36. Forest MG, Cathiard AM, Bertrand JA: Total and unbound testosterone levels in the newborn and in normal and hypogonadal children: Use of a sensitive radioimmunoassay for testosterone. J Clin Endocrinol Metab 36:1132-1142, 1973.

37. Forest MG, Cathiard AM, Bertrand JA: Evidence of testicular activity in early infancy. J Clin Endocrinol Metab 37:148-151, 1973.

38. Chaussain JL, Brijawi P, Georges P, Roger M, Donnadieu M, Job JC: Variations of serum testosterone estradiol binding globulin (TeBG) binding capacity in infants during the first year of life. Acta Paediatr 67:649-653, 1978.

39. Kärkkäinen J, Nikkari T, Ruponen S, Haahti E: Lipids of vernix caseosa. J Invest Dermatol 44:333-338, 1965.

40. Ansari MNA, Fu HC, Nicolaides N: Fatty acids of the alkane diol esters of vernix caseosa. Lipids 5:279-282, 1970.

41. Nicolaides N, Fu HC, Ansari MNA, Rice GR: The fatty acids of wax esters and sterol esters from vernix caseosa and from human skin surface lipid. Lipids 7:506-517, 1972.

42. Aly R, Maibach HI, Shinefield HR, Strauss WG: Survival of pathogenic microorganisms on human skin. J Invest Dermatol 58:205-210, 1972.

43. Aly R, Maibach HI, Rahman R, Shinefield HR, Mandel AD: Correlation of human in vivo and in vitro cutaneous antimicrobial factors. J Infect Dis 131:579-583, 1975.

44. Puhvel SM, Reisner RM: Effect of fatty acids on the growth of *Corynebacterium acnes in vitro*. J Invest Dermatol 54:48-52, 1970.

45. Ko HL, Heczko PB, Pulverer G: Differential susceptibility of *Propionibacterium acnes*, *P. granulosum* and *P. avidum* to free fatty acids. J Invest Dermatol 71:363-365, 1978.

46. Parran JJ, Brinkman RE: The effect of human skin surface lipids upon the activity of antimicrobial agents. J Invest Dermatol 45:89-92, 1965.

47. Skinner WA, Tong H, Maibach H, Khan AA, Pearson T: Repellency of skin-surface lipids of humans to mosquitoes. Science 149:305-306, 1965.

48. Skinner WA, Tong HC, Maibach HI, Skidmore D: Human skin-surface lipid fatty acids—mosquito repellents. Experientia 26:728-730, 1970.

49. Beare JM, Rook A: The newborn, in *Textbook of Dermatology*, edited by Rook A, Wilkinson DS, and Ebling, FJG. F. A. Davis, Philadelphia, 1968, p 113.

50. Prose PH: Pathologic changes in eczema. J Pediatr 66:178-199, 1965.

51. Rajka G: Surface lipid estimation on the back of the hands in atopic dermatitis. Arch Dermatol Forsch 251:43-48, 1974.

52. Mustakallio KK, Kiistala U, Piha HJ, Nieminen E: Epidermal lipids in Besnier's prurigo (atopic eczema). Ann Med Exp Fenn 45:323-345, 1967.

53. Ead RD, Fairbank RA, Cunliffe WJ: Sebum excretion rate, surface lipid composition and constitutional eczema. Clin Exp Dermatol 2:361-364, 1977.

54. Gloor M, Strack R, Geissler H, Friederich HC: Quantity and composition of skin surface lipids and alkaline-resistance in subjects with contact allergy and in healthy controls. Arch Dermatol Forsch 245:184-190, 1972.

55. Vallecchi C, Tinti P, Panconesi E: Surface lipids of healthy and eczematous skin (eczema due to occupational contact). Ital Gen Rev Dermatol 7:1-11, 1966.

56. Bessone L: Acne infantum. Chron Dermatol 3:43-67, 1972.

FUNCTION

4

A Review of Transepidermal Water Loss

DONALD R. WILSON and HOWARD MAIBACH
University of California Medical School, San Francisco, California

STRATUM CORNEUM AS A PHYSICAL BARRIER

The principal water barrier function of the epidermis resides almost entirely in the stratum corneum (SC), the thin coherent membrane of keratinized epithelial cells comprising the dead surface layer of the epidermis. The SC is 10-20 n thick on the back, arms, legs, and abdomen but 400-600 n on plantar and palmar callus [1]. The SC provides most of the mechanical strength of the epidermis. The viable epidermis, by comparison, is relatively permeable and mechanically weak [2].

The bulk of the stratum corneum appears as a uniformly good diffusion barrier regardless of depth [3,4] despite the observation that intracorneal binding forces decrease and anatomical changes take place (cells become flatter, more polygonal, exhibit less surface folding, and loose desmosomal attachments) as the cells move outward from the granular layer. The decrease in cohesive force may or may not be linear with depth [5].

The SC cells are stacked, those of different layers interdigitating somewhat, and are closely packed with all narrow intercellular spaces filled. SC cells contain polymerized keratin filaments 60-80 Å in diameter distributed in an amorphous matrix of lipid and nonfibrous protein [6].

The SC has an affinity for, and will pass, water-soluble and lipid-soluble compounds due to the inherent mosaic filament-matrix ultrastructure allowing aqueous and lipid regions to exist separately. The hydrated intracellular keratin

83

is apparently the rate-limiting diffusion media for water and completely water-soluble compounds [2]. Diffusion occurs passively down a concentration gradient. The intercellular regions of the SC contain lipid-rich amorphous material preventing it from becoming a major water diffusion route. Water apparently diffuses through intercellular regions and cell membranes without discrimination [2].

Since the SC is not simply an inert membrane material but one with an affinity for water, Fick's diffusion law for a simple membrane:

$$J_s = \frac{D(C_1 - C_2)}{\delta}$$

is modified to

$$J_s = \frac{K_m D \Delta C_s}{\delta}$$

and

$$K_p = \frac{K_m D}{\delta}$$

where

J_s = steady-state flux of water, mol cm^{-2} hr^{-1}
ΔC_s = concentration gradient of water across membrane, mol cm^{-3}
$C_1 - C_2 = \Delta C_s$
K_p = permeability constant for water, cm hr^{-1}
δ = membrane thickness, cm
$K_m = \dfrac{\text{concentration sorbed in membrane}}{\text{concentration in solution}}$, a partition coefficient
D = membrane diffusion constant for water, cm^2 sec^{-1}

J_s for water diffusing through the SC is measurable at the skin surface as transepidermal water loss (TEWL). TEWL (μg cm^{-2} hr^{-1}) $\sim J_s$ (mol cm^{-2} hr^{-1}); all factors relevant to J_s also extend to TEWL.

The concentration gradient ΔC_s, for in vivo SC, is dependent on ambient relative humidity (RH). The gradient develops through evaporation from the skin surface; ΔC_s approaches zero as the RH nears 100%.

The water concentration for a skin surface at 31°C and 40% RH is about 11.7 M. The lowest layer of the SC contains 48.3-49.4 M water [2] equal to that of the viable epidermis. The concentration gradient would consequently be about 37.2 M.

The membrane diffusion constant (D) is highly temperature dependent because the activation energies for diffusion across the SC are high [2]. The diffusion rate increases exponentially with rising temperature; so does TEWL. The effect of temperature on TEWL has been documented [7]. A skin temperature increase is implied as a possible cause for radiant heat and phototherapy elevating TEWL [8-11]. Temperature affects the partitioning coefficient (K_m) to a lesser degree.

Hydration of the SC has a special effect: the thickness (δ) and diffusion constant (D) increase; the partition coefficient (K_m) may increase or decrease depending on concentration. For water diffusion, the increases of δ and D are antagonistic, but D dominates resulting in an increase in TEWL [12].

TEWL has evolved from a measurement employed to help assess the dehydration rate of a whole infant [11] to an indicator of epidermal integrity [13,14]. As an indicator TEWL can demonstrate a difference from normal but cannot, by itself, identify the cause of a difference; K_m, D, δ, and ΔC_s must be investigated.

Sensible sweating must be eliminated during any TEWL measurement utilized in assessing stratum corneum integrity. This is easily achieved by: (1) measuring subjects (or local skin area) in a cool environment (e.g., 15°C) which will induce a skin temperature below 34°C, and (2) insuring the subject is emotionally calm (preventing sympathetic stimulation due to excitement). Sensible sweating is most completely eliminated by intracutaneous injection, iontophoresis, or topical application (facilitated by occlusion) of an atropinelike receptor site inhibitor [15,7]. Thiele and Malten [16] and Thiele et al. [15] employing Permlastic sweat prints, demonstrate that some sweating occurs on the forearm in comfortable ambient temperatures from 20 to 24°C. They suggest this sweating is not blocked by a receptor site inhibitor yet still conclude that thermoregulation of the lower forearm occurs through activation and deactivation of the sweat glands (an intrinsic skin phenomenon?). They state that water transport via the skin is not so much based on diffusion through the horny layer but occurs by diffusion and hydrodynamic flow via the sweat gland. This conflicts with the Scheuplein and Blank [2] interpretation as well as electrophysiological evidence [17].

The above work [15,16], and that of Rothman [18] and Bettley and Grice [19], give rise to the statement that insensible perspiration consists of a continuous diffusion of water through the epidermis and a slight secretion of sweat through the sweat glands. Recent work in our laboratory involving TEWL of fresh excised cadaver skin and in vivo skin in a cool environment (14°C produced shivering) suggest the exclusion of any sweating from insensible TEWL.

Inner thigh TEWL of 10 cadavers was measured at a controlled skin temperature of 30°C; forearm and back TEWL of 10 cool room subjects were measured at skin temperatures 24-31°C, but were corrected to 30°C according to a modification of Grice et al. [7]. The two TEWL groups at 30°C were tested with an unpaired data t-test resulting in no apparent difference existing between cadavers and in vivo skin. The cadaver skin was fresh and refrigerated in Hank's solution 2-4 days before use. The cold room subjects probably exhibited no thermally induced sweating as their shivering indicated effective hypothermia.

The following explanations are possible:

1. Sweating actually exists in both cadaver and in vivo skin at the same level of activity.
2. Sweating occurred only in the cadaver group (cadaver and in vivo TEWL means, 552.0 and 525.7 $g\,cm^{-2}\,hr^{-1}$, respectively) but was insignificantly effective on TEWL.
3. Sweating did not occur in cadaver or in vivo skin.

The third explanation is preferred since skin tissue rarely survives past 72 hr (death begins within 24 hr); [20] most cadaver samples were probably dead, thus preventing sweating.

No empirical evidence actually demonstrates the existence of an intrinsic thermally induced sweating reflex (lacking innervation) and visual comparison of graphic dissimilar data is the only evidence [17]. Ours implies that sweating probably plays no part in insensible water loss.

TEWL TECHNIQUES

Urine Osmolarity

Principle: Given a constant fluid intake for an infant, a change in insensible water loss will produce a directly proportional change in urine osmolarity and specific gravity.

Method: Infants are kept in incubators adjusted to maintain a rectal temperature of 37°C, and urine collection bags are applied. Bags are removed just after the infant voids and the time noted. Osmometer or refractometer measurements are taken for each void [21].

Pros
1. Osmometers and particularly refractometers are readily available in most intensive care nurseries (ICNs). A slightly curvilinear (almost linear) relationship exists between osmolarity and specific gravity; either measurement can be taken.

2. Hospital staff can easily take the measurements without specific training.
3. Procedure is effective in assessing general evaporative fluid balance of infants.

Cons

1. Insensible water loss change is only assumed to produce a proportional urine osmolarity (mmol kg^{-1}), or specific gravity (g urine g water^{-1})
2   TEWL cannot be separated from respiration water loss.

Body Weight

Principle: Insensible water loss (IWL) = insensible weight loss minus (CO_2 - O_2).

Method: Infants are placed in an incubator, temperature is controlled, RH is measured with wet and dry bulb thermometers or an electric hygrometer. Infants are weighed on scales (with an accuracy at least 0.5 g) at least every 3 hr. Spitting, sweating, or very active infants are not measured. Insensible weight loss (g m^{-2} day^{-1}) = initial body weight minus intake minus (final weight and exretia). Ten percent of weight loss occurs from the weight of CO_2 excreted minus O_2 consumed; this is ignored as a small constant error [8,10,11,22].

Pros

1. All necessary equipment is readily available in most ICNs with the exception of a RH device.
2. ICN staff can easily take necessary measurements without special training.
3. Method is effective in assessing total IWL.
4. Measurement can be continuous employing a recording balance [23].

Cons

1. Since balance sensitivities are low, the measurement period is long, hours or days.
2. TEWL is not separable from total IWL.

Closed Chamber—Weight Hygroscopic Substance

Principle: Dry hygroscopic substances absorb water vapor which can be weighed:

$$ WL = \frac{w_{after} - w_{before}}{A \, \Delta T} $$

where
  WL = water loss, g
   w = weight of substance
   A = area, cm^2
   ΔT = time interval

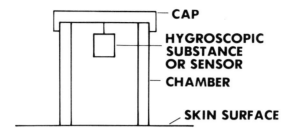

Figure 1 Closed transepidermal water loss chamber; a general design (cross-section.

Method: A glass tube of known internal diameter is attached to a skin site. A hygroscopic substance (calcium chloride, magnesium perchlorate, silica gel) is weighed and placed in the tube (Fig. 1). The capsule remains on the skin 15-30 min, after which the hygroscopic material is removed and weighed. Sensitivity increases with the area and time interval measured. To achieve a resolution of about 10% normal TEWL ($0.5 \text{ g m}^{-2} \text{ hr}^{-1}$), a weight accuracy of 0.125 is necessary. The hygroscopic material cannot become saturated during the measurement, which limits the measurement period [4,24].

Powers and Fox [25] modified the technique by filling a fritted glass (normal glass sandwich with silica gel, making a capsule) and weighing the entire unit.

Hattingh [26] stirred the chamber air with an internal fan enhancing water absorption. Lamke et al. [27] stirred the chamber air as well but replaced the hygroscopic substance with an electrohygrometer probe (similar to that in the Evaporimeter [28]). With continuous recording Lamke measured TEWL from the initial rate of vapor concentration increase within the chamber.

Pros
1. The simple capsules are easy and inexpensive to make; the procedure is simple. Units with fans and electric hygrometers are more difficult to build.
2. The measurements are taken from local skin areas and are sensitive enough for sample comparison.
3. The Lamke et al. [27] method appears the most accurate for closed chambers.

Cons
1. TEWL cannot be continuously recorded by any closed chamber method.
2. Actual TEWL is not measurable by the simple capsule method because (a) The RH of the capsule increases as the hygroscopic substance approaches saturation; this decreases ΔC_s during measurement; and (b) vapor in the chamber before the hygroscopic substance is introduced produces a higher

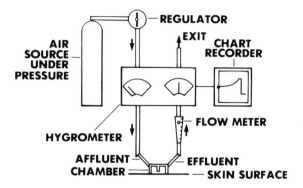

Figure 2 General design for ventilated transepidermal water loss chamber (cross-section) connected with air, source, hygrometer, flow meter, and recorder.

than normal TEWL. This variable must be measured with a control capsule and subtracted from TEWL.

Ventilated Chambers

The ventilated chamber technique, regardless of the method of water measurement, involves passing a continuous gas flow of known humidity and velocity through a sampling chamber (incubator for total infant body measurement or cup for a local skin area). The chamber effluent humidity is then measured and compared with the affluent humidity. A typical ventilated chamber system is diagrammed in Figure 2. The following equation generally applies to ventilated chamber measurements:

$$WL = F \times \frac{M}{RTA_v} (P_{H_2O(eff)} - P_{H_2O(aff)})$$

where

WL = water loss, g m^{-2} hr^{-1}

F = carrier gas flow, m^3 hr^{-1}

M = molecular weight H_2O, 18 g

R = gas constant (8.314 J mol k^{-1})

T = Temperature ($^\circ$K)

A_v = area of measurement (m^2)

P_{H_2O} = vapor pressure of effluent (eff) and affluent (aff) gas (P$_a$) [29].

WL equals TEWL if a sample chamber is placed directly on a skin site and sweating is eliminated.

Ventilated chamber techniques all suffer from a forced convection factor produced by affluent air movement over the skin site. The water diffusion gradient is increased by removal of a layer of stagnant and more humid air contacting the skin surface (boundary layer). The forced convection effect increases with affluent flow rate.

Ventilated chamber techniques are excellent for relative comparisons of TEWL providing affluent flow rate and chamber design are constant, but actual TEWL (that occurring from adjacent sites in ambient air) is never really measured.

Weight Hygroscopic Substance

Principle: Dry hygroscopic substances absorb water vapor which can be weighed.

Method: An infant in an incubator receives air at a known relative humidity, flow rate, and temperature. The air in the incubator is agitated with a fan. The affluent and effluent incubator air is sampled by drawing it through cannisters of hygroscopic magnesium perchlorate with a vacuum chamber of known volume and pressure. Once a volume of air passed through the canisters, they are weighed on a balance accurate to 1.0 mg; measuring periods are 10 min. From the affluent and effluent canister weight difference, volume of vacuum chamber, body weight (or area) of the infant, and measurement period; IWL is measured. TEWL is derived from:

$$IWL = TEWL + (CO_2 - O_2)$$

where $CO_2 - O_2 = 56$ mg kg^{-1} hr^{-1} (Zweymüller and Preining [30]).

Pros
1. RH of the affluent incubator air is measured.

Cons
1. All equipment must be fabricated.
2. Operation requires good experimental technique and much mathematical manipulation. Data collection is cumbersome.
3. The sensitivity is about the same as with the body weight technique, which is much simpler. TEWL is derived, not directly measured.
4. The forced convection factor elevates TEWL above normal.

Electrohygrometer

Principle: Lithium chloride absorbs water causing electrical resistance within the crystal to increase. The temperature required to evaporate the crystal moisture returning the resistance to baseline is proportional to RH.

Method: Air $> 11\%$ RH is passed through a sampling chamber 2 measuring 25 cm^2 of skin (producing a sensitivity of 641.7 Pa g^{-1} cm^{-2} min^{-1}). The affluent and effluent gases are measured with the electrohygrometer (two hygrometers may be used to record simultaneous and continuous measurements). The gas temperature and ambient barometric pressure are recorded. Utilization of a dry gas permits measurement of only the effluent RG [29,31].

Pros
1. Electrohygrometers are reasonably priced and are easily obtained in the United States from scientific supply houses. Sample chambers are easily constructed.
2. Hospital staff could monitor TEWL or IWL measurement; a technician could perform the necessary calculations.
3. The utilization of ambient room air permits TEWL measurement under normal RH conditions [32].

Cons
1. The chamber size (25 cm^2) is too large for convenient TEWL measurement on infants. Reduction of chamber size necessitates reduction of affluent flow rate to maintain a measurable difference in P_{H_2O}. A decrease in flow rate increases the measurement period.
2. TEWL must be manually calculated unless the hygrometer is computerized.
3. TEWL is elevated by the forced convection factor.

Thermal Conductivity Cell

Principle: The thermal conductivity of a gas mixture is changed when its composition is altered. A thermistor wire is heated by a constant current; a change in gas composition changes the wire temperature.

Method: Dry nitrogen (or nitrogen of constant humidity) is passed through a sampling chamber. The effluent water is detected by the thermal conductivity cell. The cell is very sensitive if housed in a $50°C$ environment with the flow rate constant [33].

Pros
1. A medium priced instrument obtained directly from the manufacturer.
2. The equipment is easily operated by a technician; calculation of TEWL is not difficult.
3. Instrument is sensitive.
4. Instrument effectively measures TEWL.

Cons
1. Only binary gases (e.g., nitrogen + water vapor) can be utilized.

2. TEWL must be manually calculated from RH unless computerized.
3. The binary mixture requirement excludes TEWL measurement in ambient air.
4. The forced convection factor tends to elevate TEWL.

Infrared Water Vapor Analyzer

Principle: Water vapor absorbs infrared radiation at about 1.37 m; the quantity of radiation absorbed is proportional to the concentration of water vapor.

Method: Dry nitrogen is passed into a sampling chamber (1 cm diameter) attached to the skin at a constant flow rate; the effluent water vapor is measured by the infrared analyzer. Affluent and effluent air samples are measured simultaneously with separate analysis tubes and detectors, permitting continuous measurement. With an optical bench of 1 m, a 0.1% full scale sensitivity is obtained [34].

Pros

1. A technician can easily operate the equipment and calculate TEWL.
2. Sample chamber size is small enough for premature infants; measurement is sensitive.

Cons

1. Equipment is expensive and must be ordered from the manufacturer.
2. Equipment is bulky with an optical bench of 1 m.
3. TEWL must be calculated manually unless the system is computerized.
4. The forced convection factor elevates TEWL.
5. The use of dry nitrogen artificially increases the diffusion concentration gradient, thus increasing TEWL.

Dew Point Hygrometer

Principle: RH can be determined from the ambient air temperature and dew point temperature. A light is reflected off a mirror into a photocell. Air passes over the mirror which is cooled until moisture condenses on it. The temperature of condensation is continuously recorded [35].

Pros

1. A technician can easily be trained to operate equipment and calculated TEWL.
2. Sensitivity is $\pm 1°C$ over the dew point range -60 to $+70°C$.
3. TEWL is measurable in ambient RH.

Cons

1. Instrument is only available from the United Kingdom.

2. TEWL must be calculated manually unless computerized.
3. Since dew point temperature is recorded, RH must be calculated.
4. The forced convection factor elevates TEWL.

Electrolytic Water Vapor Analyzer

Principle: Phosphorus pentoxide is hygroscopic and

$$P_2O_5 + 3H_2O \rightarrow 2\,H_3PO_4$$

An electrical current passing through the substance between platinum electrodes reverses the equation. The amount of current is proportional to the
amount of water in the system.

Method: Dry nitrogen gas is passed through a sampling chamber (0.8-1.8 cm
in diameter) attached or hand-held on a skin site; gas flow is 100 cm^3 min^{-1}. The
effluent water is measured by the analyzer in parts per million (ppm) [13,15,16,
36,37]. Sensitivity is about 1 ppm.

Pros
1. Equipment is moderately priced and available in the United States.
2. A technician can easily be trained to take ppm measurements and calculate
   TEWL.
3. The small chamber size permits measurement of premature infants.
4. The 30 sec time constant of the cell permits continuous measurement of
   TEWL providing fluctuation durations are at least several minutes.

Cons
1. TEWL must be manually calculated from ppm unless the system is computerized.
2. While the operation is simple, the total time required for a single measurement
   is 5-15 min depending on circumstances. The baseline humidity of the affluent gas takes several hours to stabilize. Without stabilization baseline drift
   must be calculated.
3. Since only low humidities $\leqslant$ 1000 ppm (equivalent to 3.29% RH at 25°C) are
   directly measurable, the effluent gas must be split and only a fraction measured or the skin surface area must be reduced bring ppm back on scale. Both
   adjustments are awkward, especially the latter.
4. The necessity of employing dry nitrogen falsely increases the water diffusion
   concentration gradient across the skin; consequently TEWL are artificially
   high.
5. The forced convection factor elevates TEWL above normal.

Dielectric Permittivity

Principle: The degree of dielectric permittivity of a water vapor-air mixture filling a resonant cavity is a function of the amount of water vapor present.

Method: Atmospheric air is pumped at $333.3 \text{ cm}^3 \text{ min}^{-1}$ through a sample chamber attached to a skin site measuring 30 cm^2. Air is pumped through a completely closed chamber (reference) simultaneously. The effluent air from both chambers pass to respective resonance cavities containing 8.5 GHz electromagnetic radiation. The resonance curves are plotted from the detectors of each cavity, and any frequency difference (proportional to water content difference) is calculated by an electronic clock. From 10-1000 measurements are taken and averages computed internally. Measurements occur in about 2 min after sample chamber attachment. The apparatus is calibrated with a box of accurately weighed water establishing a direct relationship between frequency shift and water loss [38].

Pros
1. A technician should be able to operate equipment and take measurements.
2. Technique is ultrasensitive.
3. TEWL is directly measured.
4. Measurements are made in 2 min and continuous measurements are possible.
5. TEWL is measurable in ambient RH.

Cons
1. The apparatus is not commercially available.
2. Sample chamber size is presently too large for convenient measurement of infants (area reduction seems possible).
3. The affluent flow rate is three times higher than with the electrolytic analyzer; the forced convection factor is proportionally greater.

Open Chamber: Water Evaporation Gradient

Principle: Without forced convection, a boundary layer of air develops on the skin with a water gradient developed from skin surface and atmospheric humidity; the boundary layer is about 1 cm high. TEWL can be derived from the distribution of vapor pressure and temperature of this layer.

$$\text{TEWL} (\text{g m}^{-2} \text{ h}^{-1}) = D' \frac{dP}{dx}$$

where
$$D' = \text{constant } 0.670 \times 10^{-3} \text{ g} (\text{mhP}_a^{-1})$$

$$\frac{dP}{dx} = \text{vapor pressure gradient (Pa m}^{-1})$$

Method: The instrument (ServoMed Evaporimeter) is capable of measuring RH (%), P_{H_2O} (mmHg), and evaporation water loss (g m^{-2} hr^{-1}). The evaporimeter probe contains two humidity sensors coated with an organic polymer dielectrically sensitive to humidity stacked vertically 6 mm apart. Each sensor is coupled with a thermistor and thus are enclosed in a Teflon cylinder (1 cm in diameter) open at both ends (Fig. 3). The probe is held against the skin surface with the sensors oriented parallel to the vapor gradient of the boundary layer. The boundary layer stabilizes within the cylinder in 2-15 min. Air turbulence over the exposed cylinder end must be minimized to prevent destruction of the vapor gradient. The sensor sensitivity is about 9.0 Pa g^{-1} m^{-1} hr [29].

Pros
1. Hospital staff or technicians can easily use the Evaporimeter.
2. 0.1 g m^{-2} hr^{-1} water loss is the smallest unit measurable, sufficient for dermatology research.
3. RH, P_{H_2O}, and evaporation rate values are computed internally by the instrument.
4. Measurement accuracy is not dependent on the skin area measured. A small cylinder can be utilized for premature infants.
5. TEWL is measurable in ambient RH.
6. There is no forced convection factor.

Cons
1. Instrument is only made in Sweden.
2. Warm-up time is 1 hr.
3. Local air currents over skin surface do affect measurement and must be controlled.
4. RH fluctuations affect measurement and should be controlled experimentally.
5. Skin temperature must be measured separately.

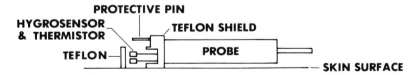

Figure 3   Open transepidermal water loss chamber (Evaporimeter). Hygrosensors coupled with thermistors measure water evaporation at the skin surface. Cross-section through Teflon shield shows sensor arrangement.

Electromagnetic Probe

Principle: The rotation of liquid water in an electromagnetic field absorbs energy and produces a frequency shift. The degree of electromagnetic field alteration is proportional to water concentration.

Method: Electromagnetic radiation is generated in a wave guide probe (resonance cavity) consisting of a coaxial cable which terminates in a small slit. The slit width limits the field depth of penetration. Presently 90% of the field penetrates approximately 3 μm. The probe is touched on the skin surface and the stratum corneum water content is measured in –mV within 1 sec. MV are directly converted to % water content. The probe occludes TEWL during the measurement of percentage water content and the water content increases with time. The rate of hydration under the probe is proportional to TEWL if measured as soon as possible after probe contact. Jacques [39] describes an early version of the electromagnetic probe.

Pros
1. The probe is extremely simple to use and can probably be employed by hospital staff on premature infants.
2. Accuracy is ± 1% water content.
3. Percentage water content and TEWL are obtained faster than with any other method.
4. Continuous measurement of TEWL is not possible but the high sampling rate (30-60/hr) offsets this inconvenience.
5. There is no forced convection factor.

Cons
1. Equipment cannot be purchased; it is experimental.
2. Instrument adjustment and calibration require training. The best radiation frequency is not yet standardized.
3. The accuracy of TEWL measurement is unknown; however, the values fall within those of other instruments.
4. Some phenomena occur during measurement which are not presently explainable; they may affect measurement and need investigation (e.g., pressure at which probe is applied to the skin).

CONCLUSION

Leveque et al. [38] proposed that the following characteristics should be met with the best TEWL measurement system:

1. The device should not alter the physical and chemical properties of the SC.

2. The surface area measured should not be too large or small.
3. Measurements should be differential (both temporal and spacial) permitting recording of minute variations.
4. Measurement should take no more than 2 or 3 min to avoid stressing the infant.

The best TEWL method employed on infants in the future may be the electromagnetic probe since it is small, measurements are fast, and technique is simple. Conditions 2, 3, and 4 are met with the probe. Condition 1 needs thorough investigation since TEWL is taken by momentarily occluding the skin with the probe; the occlusion effect on the stratum corneum water concentration gradient must be known.

The best commercially available TEWL instrument is the Evaporimeter by ServoMed, Sweden. All of Leveque et al.'s conditions are met. Condition 4 is met most of the time; air disturbances over the measuring cylinder destroy the boundary layer and additional time is sometimes needed for the TEWL measurement to stabilize.

The dielectric permittivity instrument of Leveque et al. [38] may well be the next best TEWL instrument for infant measurement if the sample chamber can be made smaller and the flow rate slower. TEWL readings are obtained consistently in 2-3 min, the measurement is sensitive, and is made with ambient RH. The instrument, however, is not yet commercially available.

The electrolytic water vapor analyzer remains as a moderately priced TEWL method despite the exposure of the skin to dry nitrogen, an affluent flow rate of 100 cm^3/min, a measurement time of 5-15 min, and a 1-2 hr drying down time before use. It is excellent for comparative studies where true TEWL is not required and serves well testing moisturizer effectiveness [37].

SUMMARY

TEWL, the insensible flux of water through the stratum corneum, is directly measurable from local skin sites with closed chamber, ventilated chamber, and open chamber-evaporation gradient techniques. The closed chamber methods are incapable of continuous measurement and tend to occlude the skin, changing its permeability characteristics during measurement. Ventilated chambers provide continuous TEWL [30], but it is usually elevated due to destruction of the boundary layer as affluent air passes over the skin site. The use of dry nitrogen in many ventilated chamber techniques (e.g., electrolytic and infrared analyzers and thermal conductivity cell) further elevates TEWL by increasing the water concentration gradient across the skin. The open chamber-evaporation gradient method (the best commercially available) provides continuous measurement in ambient air with little alteration of the vapor boundary layer overlying the skin. Measurements are made in 2-5 min; TEWL (evaporation rate) is displayed on the machine face.

REFERENCES

1. Rushmer RF, Buettner KJK, Short JM, Odland GF: The skin. Science 154: 343-348, 1966.
2. Scheuplain RJ, Blank IH: Permeability of the skin. Physiol Rev 51:702-747, 1971.
3. Blank IH: Further observations on factors which influence the water content of the stratum corneum. J Invest Dermatol 21:259-269, 1953.
4. Monash S, Blank H: Location and reformation of the epithelial barrier to water vapor. Arch Dermatol 78:710-714, 1958.
5. King CS, Barton SP, Nichols S, Marks R: The changes in properties of the stratum corneum as a function of depth. Br J Dermatol 100:165-172, 1979.
6. Brady I: The ultrastructure of the tonofibrils in the keratinization process of normal human epidermis. J Ultrastruct Res 4:264-297, 1960.
7. Grice K, Sattar H, Sharrat M, Baker H: Skin temperature and transepidermal water loss. J Invest Dermatol 57:108, 1971.
8. Williams PR, Oh W: Effects of radiant warmer on insensible water loss in newborn infants. Am J Dis Child 128:511-514, 1974.
9. Bell EF, Nerdich GA, Cashore WJ, Oh W: Combined effect of radiant warmer and phototherapy on insensible water loss in low-birth weight infants. J Pediatr 94:810-813, 1979.
10. Wu PYK, Hodgman JE: Insensible water loss in pre-term infants: Changes with postnatal development and non-ionizing radiant energy. Pediatrics 54: 704-712, 1974.
11. Fanaroff AA, Wald M, Gruber HS, Klaus MH: Insensible water loss in low birth weight infants. Pediatrics 50:236-245, 1972.
12. Dugard PH: Skin permeability theory in relation to measurements of percutaneous absorption in toxicology, in *Dermatotoxicology and Pharmacology*, edited by Marzulli FN and Maibach HI. Hemisphere, Washington, D.C., p 567.
13. Cunico RL, Maibach HI, Khan H, Bloom E: Skin barrier properties in the newborn: Transepidermal water loss and carbon dioxide emission rates. Biol Neonate 32:177-182, 1977.
14. Wilson DR, Maibach HI: Transepidermal water loss in vivo premature and term infants. Biol Neonate 37:180-185, 1980.
15. Thiele FAJ, Hemels HGWM, Malten KE: Skin temperature and water loss by skin. Trans St. John's Hosp Dermatol Soc 58:218-223, 1972.
16. Thiele FAJ, Malten KE: Insensible water loss: The intersubject variation related to skin temperature, forearm circumference, and sweat gland activity. Trans St John's Hosp Dermatol Soc 58:199-217, 1972.

17. Montagna W, Ellis RA, Silver AF: *Advances in Biology of Skin, Vol. 3.* Pergamon Press, New York, 1962, p 266.
18. Rothman S: *Physiology and Biochemistry of the Skin.* University of Chicago Press, Chicago, 1954, p 239.
19. Bettley FR, Grice KA: A method for measuring the transepidermal water loss and a means of inactivating sweat glands. Br J Dermatol 77:627-638, 1965.
20. Elias P: Veterans Hospital, San Francisco, personal communication, 1980.
21. Jones RWA, Rochefort MJ, Baum JD: Increased insensible water in newborn infants nursed under radiant heaters. Br Med J 2:1347-1350, 1976.
22. Yeh TF, Amma P, Lilien LD, Baccaro MM, Malwynshyn J, Pyati S, Pildes RS: Reduction of insensible water loss in premature infants under the radiant warmer. J Pediatr 94:651-653, 1979.
23. Brebner DF, Kerslake DM, Waddell JL: The diffusion of water vapor through human skin. J Physiol 132:225-231, 1956.
24. Shahidullah M, Raffle EJ, Frain-Bell W: Insensible water loss in dermatitis. Br J Dermatol 79:589-597, 1967.
25. Powers DH, Fox C: A study of the effect of cosmetic ingredients, creams, and lotions on the rate of moisture loss from the skin. Toilet Goods Assoc Proc Sci Section 28:21-26, 1957.
26. Hattingh J: The influence of skin temperature, environmental temperature, and relative humidity on transepidermal water loss. Acta Dermatovener 52:438-440, 1972.
27. Lamke L-O, Nilsson GE, Reithner HL: Water loss by evaporation from the abdominal cavity during surgery. Acta Chir Scand 143:279-284, 1977.
28. Hammarlund K, Nilsson GE, Oberg PA, Sedin G: Transepidermal water loss in newborn infants. Acta Paediatr Scand 66:553-562, 1977.
29. Nilsson GE, Oberg PA: Measurement of evaporative water loss: Methods and clinical applications, in *Non-invasive Physiological Measurements*, edited by Rolfe P. Academic Press, London, 1979, p 349.
30. Zweymuller E, Preining O: The insensible water loss of the newborn infant. Acta Paediatr Scand [Suppl] 205:5-29, 1970.
31. Baker H, Kligman AM: Measurement of transepidermal water loss by electrical hygrometry. Arch Dermatol 96:441-452, 1967.
32. Reinhardt H, Brenneisen G: A new method of measuring skin humidity. J Appl Phys 41:256-258, 1976.
33. Spruit D: Measurement of the water vapor loss from human skin by a thermal conductivity cell. J Appl Physiol 23:994-997, 1967.
34. Foster KG, Hey EN, Katz G: The response of the sweat glands of the newborn baby to thermal stimuli and to intradermal acetylcholine. J Physiol 203:13-29, 1969.
35. Brengelmann GL, McKoog M, Rowell LB: Use of dew-point detection for quantitative measurement of sweating rate. J Appl Physiol 39:498-502, 1975.
36. Spruit D, Malten KE: Epidermal water-barrier formation after stripping of normal skin. J Invest Dermatol 45:6-14, 1965.

37. Rietschel RL: A skin moisturization assay. J Soc Cosmet Chem 30:369-373, 1979.
38. Leveque JL, Garson JC, de Rigal J: Transepidermal water loss from dry and normal skin. J Soc Cosmet Chem 30:333-343, 1979.
39. Jacques SL: A linear measurement of the water content of the stratum corneum of human skin using a microwave probe. IEEE Engineering in Medicine and Biology Society, 1st Annual Conference, 1979.

5

An In Vivo Comparison of Skin Barrier Function

DONALD R. WILSON and HOWARD MAIBACH
University of California Medical School, San Francisco, California

The relative permeability of neonatal skin to chemicals is an important consideration in light of studies demonstrating the deleterious effects of topically applied
compounds such as aniline dyes [1], pentachlorophenol [2], corticosteroids [3],
and hexachlorophene [4]. Increased skin permeability in preterm infants was
suggested by Nachman and Esterly [5] after observing the blanching response to
topically applied Neo-Synephrine. They noted a rapid response in premature infants but no response in most mature infants. Kopelman [6] suggested that the
relative penetration of hexachlorophene in preterm infants was related to postnatal age.

Baker and Kligman [7], noted that measurement of transepidermal water loss
(TEWL) from the surface of anhidrotic skin provides a sensitive index of one
specific epidermal function, the barrier function. Furthermore, this parameter
may have a relationship to the permeability of the stratum corneum for other
compounds, particularly polar compounds. Comparison of TEWL in the newborn and adult yields information about the maturity of the physical barrier in
the newborn.

The assessment of skin barrier function in newborn premature-term infants
and adults as indicated by TEWL involved two studies: change of TEWL with
gestational age in premature infants [8] and comparison of term infant with
adult TEWL [9].

TEWL VERSUS GESTATIONAL AGE IN PREMATURE INFANTS

Past research left newborn premature infant TEWL in dispute. Parmely and Seeds [10] studied the isotopic water permeability of fetal skin in vitro between 12 and 24 weeks of gestational age (GA). Unkeratinized skin of fetuses of 12-18 weeks GA had permeabilities similar to amnion and chorion laeve; partially and well-keratinized skin from fetuses of 18-24 weeks GA showed little or no water permeability. The degree of keratinization appeared to determine the water permeability.

Since fetal skin develops a histologically apparent stratum corneum by 25 weeks GA [11], premature infants by 26-28 weeks GA presumably would have TEWL comparable to a term infant. Fanaroff et al. [12] presented contrary in vivo evidence: 10 infants less than 32 weeks GA lost > 2.5 g kg^{-1} hr^{-1}, considerably higher than previously reported. These values were derived from body weight losses measured with a sensitive balance, and constituting the sum of respiratory and transepidermal water loss. An increased metabolic rate was discounted as a possible factor; thinner epidermis, increased water content, and increased permeability were suggested skin factors producing this large water loss.

TEWL of local skin sites was measured with GA in infants 26-41 weeks GA to test the above assumptions and yield information on the development of the physical skin barrier.

Materials and Methods

TEWL measurements were taken on 28 infants 2-9 days old and from 26-41 weeks GA (body weights 630-4100 g at measurement). Premature infants (less than 37 weeks GA) were in temperature-controlled isolettes or open cribs with or without radiant heat or bililights; several were under heat shields or plastic (Saran) wrap which was removed before measurement. Some infants were on respirators or supplimentary O_2; several had cranial or umbilical intravenous catheters. All premature infants had attached electrocardiogram (ECG) electrodes; some were diapered.

Normal term infants were in open cribs at room temperature, wrapped in blankets, and diapered. These were partially removed for most measurements. All infants were estimated to be average for gestational age from body weight and length measurements.

TEWL was measured on the upper arm, chest, abdomen, upper and lower back, and/or thigh using a Meeco electrolytic water analyzer. Dry nitrogen gas (99.9%) was passed through a molecular sieve to reduce water content and into a 1.8 cm^2 aperture sampling cup at a rate of 100 cm^3 min^{-1}. The cup, fitted with a thermistor for simultaneous measurement of skin temperature, was hand-held over the measuring site with enough pressure to maintain nitrogen flow by preventing leaks.

The sample gas exited the cup and passed to the water analyzer. Strip chart recordings of TEWL in parts per million ($TEWL_{ppm}$) were taken.

The measuring procedure involved placing the sample cup on a skin site and recording $TEWL_{ppm}$ with time until a slope of zero was obtained. The level $TEWL_{ppm}$ minus the residual water at baseline provided a true $TEWL_{ppm}$ used for calculation. $TEWL_{ppm}$ was converted to TEWL in micrograms per square centimeter per hour ($TEWL_{\mu g\ cm^{-2}hr^{-1}}$) as follows:

$$TEWL_{\mu g\ cm^{-2}hr^{-1}} = \frac{TEWL_{ppm}\,(7.3617 \times 10^{-2}\ \mu g\ min^{-1})(60\ min)}{1.8\ cm^2}$$

where $7.3617\ \mu g\ min^{-1}$ = weight of water vapor in air sample flowing at 100 cm/min, $1.8\ cm^2$ = aperture area of cup, and 60 min = 1 hr.

Results

$TEWL_{g\ cm^{-2}hr^{-1}}$ measurements versus respective GA were plotted (Fig. 1). The points for infants between 31 and 41 weeks GA appear randomly scattered; those of lower GA infants appear to be higher. There is a trend towards increased TEWL with lower GA.

A linear regression analysis (model 1, 1 independent variable) [13] provided a regression coefficient of $-97.25\ \mu g\ cm^{-2}\ hr^{-1}$. The regression line runs through the y intercept $4186.0\ \mu g\ cm^{-2}\ hr^{-1}$ and grand mean point $34.6\ \bar{x}$, $815.1\ \bar{y}$ (Fig. 1). With a calculated F of 39.9 and 91 degrees of freedom (error mean square), the regression coefficient is highly significant, $P < 0.01$.

A test for regression linearity [13] was performed to determine how well the points on the figure fit a straight line. The calculated F of 13.07 with 12 degrees of freedom for deviation from linearity and 79 degrees of freedom for 'within groups' is greater than 2.5, the F associated with 0.01 probability. The points on the figure appear to differ highly significantly from a linear regression.

Infants between 27 and 29 weeks GA apparently have greater TEWL than the others as indicated by an overall F test ($P < 0.01$). A dividing line separating high TEWL from lower should possibly be drawn through the 29 week GA group.

TERM INFANT VERSUS ADULT TEWL

TEWL was measured from local skin sites in term newborn infants and adults to assess similarity in skin barrier function.

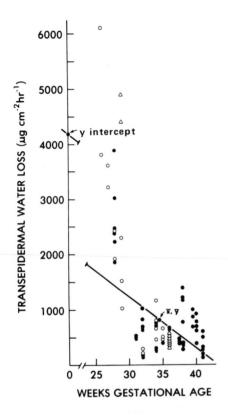

Figure 1 Transepidermal water loss relative to gestational age. Regression line shown running through y intercept and grand mean point $\bar{x}, \bar{y}$. X axis is abbreviated. $\circ$, Bililight; $\bullet$, non-bililight; $\triangle$, radiant heat infants (Adapted from Ref. 8).

Material and Methods

Subjects: Healthy term infants 3-43 weeks gestational age, were measured 1-3 days after birth, after informed parental consent was obtained. Birth weights ranged from 2,275 to 4,506 g. TEWL was measured on the volar aspect of the forearm. Infants were in open cribs and receiving no special treatment. Infants has usually been bathed 6-10 hr before measurements. Of 75 infants studied, seven were considered small for gestational age (SGA). These infants were two or more standard deviations below the mean weight for their particular gestational age.

Adult subjects sat quietly for 15-20 min before TEWL measurement. While TEWL measurements were being made on the volar aspect of one forearm. simultaneous measurements were performed on the opposite arm. In a few cases, high widely fluctuating TEWL values were observed and were undoubtedly due to sweating. Values were only recorded when readings had stabilized.

Rabbits: In a parallel study, newborn rabbits were compared to adult rabbits. During measurements, newborn rabbits were housed in a temperature-controlled environment to maintain skin temperature. Such housing was necessary because newborns were unable to maintain a skin temperature more than a few degrees above room temperature. The average skin temperature for both groups was roughly 36°C. Adult rabbits were clipped carefully, avoiding abrasion of the skin. TEWL was measured using a Meeco electrolytic water analyzer.

Results

Human: At approximately 23°C, the adults had a higher TEWL (0.387 ± 0.152 mg cm^{-2} hr^{-1} (Table 1, p = 0.046). Using an empirical formula derived by Grice et al. [14] to compare the values at a standard skin temperature, we normalized the values (Table 2). With these 'corrected' values, the results were similar to adults (0.336 ± 0.154 mg cm^{-2} hr^{-1}) (Table 2, P = 0.008). Values of SGA infants were no different from the remaining population.

Both skin and environmental temperature play a role in governing the magnitude of TEWL. The effect of changes in the environmental temperature on TEWL measurements is shown in Table 3. These values were not corrected for skin temperature.

Rabbits: In a parallel study with rabbits, TEWL measurements on 18 adults averaged 0.432 ± 0.202 mg cm^{-2} hr^{-1} and the average TEWL value for 36 newborn rabbits was 0.391 ± 0.157 mg cm^{-2} hr^{-1}. The difference between these groups was not significant.

Table 1 Transepidermal Water Loss

	Adults	Neonates
n	30	22
$\bar{x}$, mg cm^{-2} hr^{-1}	0.387	0.313
SD, mg cm^{-2} hr^{-1}	0.152	0.091
ST, °C	32.7	33.3

Average room temperature = 23.3°C; Relative humidity = 50%; P = 0.047.

n, number of observations; $\bar{x}$, mean; SD, standard deviation; ST, skin temperature.

Source: Ref. 9.

Table 2 Comparison of Corrected TEWL Values

	Adults	Neonates
n	30	22
$\bar{x}$, mg cm^{-2} hr^{-1}	0.336	0.241
SD, mg cm^{-2} hr^{-1}	0.154	0.063
	P = 0.008	

Values corrected to 32°C following Grice et al. [13].

n, number of observations; $\bar{x}$, mean; 50, standard deviation.

Source: Ref. 9.

Table 3 Newborn TEWL at Two Environmental Temperatures (No Skin Temperature Correction)

	Group 1	Group 2
n	22	35
$\bar{x}$, mg cm^{-2} hr^{-1}	0.313	0.460
SD, mg cm^{-2} hr^{-1}	0.091	0.121
RT, °C	23.3	26.3
ST, °C	33.3	34.1
	P < 0.005	

n, number of observations; $\bar{x}$, mean; SD, standard deviation; RT, room temperature; ST, skin temperature.

Source: Ref. 9.

DISCUSSION

The premature infant measurements suggested that infants 29 weeks or less (mean birth weight for 29 weeks: 1250 ± 350 g SD) have significantly greater TEWL in vivo than older GA premature infants. Older premature infants have insignificantly different TEWL from normal term infants. Newborn term infant TEWL measurements of the forearm appeared about 20% lower than those of adult forearms.

The premature results (direct TEWL measurements) agree with Fanaroff et al. [12] who demonstrated a significant difference in total insensible water loss between infants (not under heat shields) of birth weights 695-1800 g. This also agrees with Fisher [15] who demonstrated in vitro that premature infants 26-30 weeks GA have highly significantly different cutaneous permeability coefficients for ^3H_2O from those of full term infants, i.e., 37-40 weeks.

Partial agreement exists with Nachman and Esterly [16] who observed an inverse relationship between blanching response to Neo-Synephrine and infant GA, suggesting that the blanching response time reflected the degree of epidermal maturity, particularly of the stratum corneum. They noted blanching differences between their 28-34, 35-37, and 38-42 week GA groups, while our TEWL varied inversely with GA only up to 29 weeks; no difference appeared thereafter.

The discrepancy may be explained as follows: normal TEWL may occur during tape stripping recovery with the development of a parakeratotic layer of cells instead of normal stratum corneum [17]. Electron microscopic examination by Ericksson and Lamke [18] suggested these were immature corneum cells. The drying of the exposed cell layers probably reduced the diffusion constant [19] to a degree resulting in normal TEWL. This phenomenon possibly occurred in the dry immature stratum corneum of premature infants.

The term infant-adult TEWL measurements of the forearm were in excellent agreement with those estimated from the total body by Wildnauer and Kennedy [20].

Basically, two factors, eccrine activity (sweating) and permeability, determine the magnitude of TEWL.

Thermally activated sweating probably was not a significant variable in our study. Adults seem to sweat actively when the skin temperature reaches 34°C and ambient temperature is 32.3°C [15], but full-term infants who are able to sweat 24 hr after birth have thermal thresholds above that of adults throughout the newborn period [1]. Green and Behrendt [21] noted that local heating of full-sized neonates with a disk 15 mm in diameter for 10 min at temperatures of 38.5-38.8°C produced no sweating. They selected a standard disk temperature of 41.5 ± 0.3°C and tested infants ranging from 28 to 42 weeks for a sweating response; infants below 35 weeks generally failed to sweat; those above did. Their study indicates that newborn infants have a limited capacity to respond to local thermal stimulation. Heating was of longer duration and greater intensity than in adults to elicit sweating, and a considerable proportion of mature neonates and an even higher percentage of premature infants failed to respond at all. Considering the relatively low environmental temperatures, thermally induced sweating is probably insignificant.

Quantitative evidence of sweating deficiency in newborns, especially low-birth-weight infants, is provided by Foster et al. [22]. After stimulation with an intradermal injection of acetylcholine, newborns showed a much larger number of active sweat glands per unit area than adults, but a lower mean peak sweat rate. Foster et al. also substantiated the idea that premature infants respond poorly or not at all to a thermal stimulus and that term infants show only a modest response to the same stimulus.

Emotional sweating in infants is usually associated with body activity and crying. Since active and crying infants could not be measured because their movements allowed atmospheric air into the sampling cup; emotional sweating may be an insignificant variable in the present study.

In this study infants measured in a room at 26.3°C showed a low and constant TEWL. Adult TEWL values at this temperature were much higher (data not shown) and fluctuated over a larger range, undoubtedly due to sweating. The difference between newborn and adult TEWL values may be a result of a decreased eccrine response to thermal stimulus. Active sweating may have inadvertently been measured in the above adults even though measurements were made on stable portions of the water loss trace after possible sweating episodes had past.

The possibility of sweating in adult skin makes any discussion of permeability difference between newborns and adults inconclusive. Recent measurements, however, of 10 adults less inclined to sweat and 13 term newborns substantiate a significant difference between TEWL. The newborns were measured as above on the forearms, abdomen, and buttocks at room temperature (23-25°C); the adults were measured on forearm and back in a room at 14°C which inhibited thermally induced sweating (normal and atropine sulfate-inhibited sites produced similar TEWL). The data are shown in Table 4. Since no skin region variation existed within infant or adult TEWL, individual TEWL were not averaged giving sample sizes of 39 and 41 for infant and adults, respectively. TEWL was corrected to 30°C removing variation due to skin temperature; the equation of Grice et al. [14] was employed but modified with a slope 0.036 (common log TEWL $°C^{-1}$) developed in our laboratory.

Table 4 Newborn Term Infant TEWL Versus Sweat-Inhibited Adult

	Infants	Adults
n	39	41
$\bar{x}$	401.9[a]	520.3[a]
SD	139.1	180.3
ST (°C)	33.7	28.8
	P = 0.002	

[a]TEWL corrected to a skin temperature of 30°C.

n, number of observations; $\bar{x}$, mean; SD, standard deviation; ST, skin temperature.

The adult mean was 22.9% greater than the infant; the difference was highly significant (P = 0.002).

The new TEWL results involving sweat inhibited adults substantiate the previous findings and make more apparent the possibility of newborn infant skin possessing less water permeability.

The premature data show that infants of approximately 28 weeks have a less efficient barrier to water than older GA infants, and the term infant-adult data show that term infants appear to have a more effective stratum corneum than adults. Although there is no known direct correlation between skin permeability to water leaving the body and chemicals entering, we wonder if infants approximately 28 weeks have increased permeability to chemicals. Clinical judgement might indicate prudence in exposing these infants to topically applied chemicals until this is clarified.

SUMMARY

Premature infants 29 weeks or younger have significantly greater TEWL in vivo than older GA premature infants. Older premature and term infants have similar TEWL. The negative correlation of TEWL with GA is not linear; drying of enough immature corneum cells producing a normal term infant water diffusion constant by 29 weeks is a possible cause.

Forearm TEWL of newborn term infants is approximately 20% lower than that of adults. With TEWL corrected for skin temperature and adult thermal sweating controlled, the difference appears generated by the physical characteristics of stratum corneum.

REFERENCES

1. Kagan BM, Mirman B, Calvin J, Lundeen E: Cyanosis in premature infants due to aniline dye intoxication. J Pediat 34:574, 1949.
2. Armstrong RW, Eichner ER, Klein DE, Barthel WR, Bennet JV, Jonsson V, Bruce H, Loveless LE: Pentachlorophenol poisoning in a nursery for newborn infants. II. Epidemiologic and toxicology studies. J Pediat 75:317, 1969.
3. Keipert JA: The absorption of topical corticosteroids, with particular reference to percutaneous absorption in infancy and childhood. Med J Aust i: 1021, 1971.
4. Kimbrough RD: Review of the toxicity of hexachlorophene. Arch Environ Health 23:119, 1971.
5. Nachman RL, Esterly NB: Increased skin permeability in preterm infants. J Pediatr 79:628, 1971.
6. Kopelman AR: Cutaneous abosrption of hexachlorophene in low-birth weight infants. J Pediatr 82:972, 1973.

7. Baker HB, Kligman AM: Measurement of transepidermal water loss by electrical hygrometry. Arch Dermatol 96:441, 1967.
8. Wilson DR, Maibach HI: Transepidermal water loss in vivo premature and term infants. Biol Neonate 37:180-185, 1980.
9. Cunico RL, Maibach HI, Kahn, H, Bloom E: Skin barrier properties in the newborn; transepidermal water loss and carbon dioxide emission rates. Biol Neonate 32:177-182, 1977.
10. Parmley TH, Seeds AE: Fetal skin permeability to isotopic water (THO) in early pregnancy. Am J Obstet Gynecol 108:128, 1970.
11. Hashimoto K, Gross BG, DiBella RJ, Lever WF: The ultrastructure of the skin of human embryos. J Invest Dermatol 47:317-335, 1966.
12. Fanaroff AA, Wald M, Gruber HS, Klaus MH: Insensible water loss in low birth weight infants. Pediatrics 50:236-245, 1972.
13. Woolf CM: *Principles of Biometry*. Van Nostrand, Princeton, N.J., 1968, p. 359.
14. Grice K, Sattar H, Sharrat M, Baker H: Skin temperature and transepidermal water loss. J Invest Dermatol 57:108, 1971.
15. Fisher L: In vitro studies on the permeability of infant skin to water. (In preparation).
16. Nachman RL, Esterly NB: Increased skin permeability in pre-term infants. J Pediatr 79:628-632, 1971.
17. Monash S, Blank H: Location and reformation of the epithelial barrier to water vapor. Arch Dermatol 78:710-714, 1958.
18. Eriksson G, Lamke L: Regeneration of human epidermal surface water barrier function after stripping. Acta Dermatovener (Stockh) 51:169-178, 1971.
19. Scheuplein RJ, Blank IH: Permeability of the skin. Physiol Rev 51:702-742, 1971.
20. Wildnauer RH, Kennedy R: Transepidermal water loss of human newborns. J Invest Dermatol 54:483-486, 1970.
21. Green M, Behrendt H: Sweating responses of neonates to local thermal stimulation. Am J Dis Child 125:20-25, 1973.
22. Foster KG, Hey EN, Katz G: The response of the sweat glands of the newborn baby to thermal stimuli and to introdermal acetylcholine. J Physiol (Lond) 203:13, 1969.

6

Carbon Dioxide Emission Rate in the Newborn

DONALD R. WILSON and HOWARD MAIBACH
University of California Medical School, San Francisco, California

Emission of carbon dioxide from the skin was demonstrated in 1851 by Gerlach. Later, more extensive studies were performed by Shaw et al. [1] and Shaw and Messer [2]. Frame et al. [3] measured carbon dioxide emission rates (CDER) on the forearm and hand of adults. They reported an average forearm CDER of 34 nl cm^{-2} min^{-1} and an average hand CDER of 46 nl cm^{-2} min^{-1}. They showed an increased CDER after vigorous exercise or after wetting the skin. Thiele and Kempen [4] showed that CDER closely follows the water loss rate after chemically induced sweating. They also noted CDER after damaging the stratum corneum. CDER can therefore be a reflection of skin barrier efficiency.

Comparison of CDER in newborns with those in adults will yield information about the maturity of the physical barrier in the newborn as well as about eccrine activity.

MATERIAL AND METHODS

Healthy term infants, 37-43 weeks of gestational age, were measured 1-3 days after birth, after informed parental consent was obtained. Birth weights ranged from 2275 to 4506 g.

CDER was measured on the upper back in infants and forearm in adults. Infants were in open cribs and receiving no special treatment. Infants had usually

This chapter was adapted from Biol Neonate 32:117-182, 1977.

been bathed 6-10 hr before measurements were begun. Of 75 infants studied, seven were considered small for gestational age (SGA). These infants were 2 or more standard deviations below the mean weight for their particular gestational age.

Adult subjects sat quietly for 15-20 min while a measurable steady-state CDER developed. CDER was measured with a Luft-type infrared analyzer similar to that described by Thiele and Kempen [4]. By employing appropriately filled reference and filter cells, the instrument can be made to respond specifically to changes in CO_2 concentrations in the ppm range. Ultrahigh purity nitrogen was directed into a 9.6 cm^2 plexiglass sampling cup at a flow rate of 50 cm^3 min^{-1}, then through the sample cell of the infrared analyzer. Instrument calibration was performed by passing standard CO_2/N_2 mixtures through the sample cell at a rate of 50 cm^3 min^{-1}. Skin temperature measurements were made with a Yellow Springs telethermometer.

RESULTS

The data for CDER showed the adults were higher (23.1 ± 6.8 nl cm^{-2} min^{-1}) than the neonates (21.8 ± 5.4 nl cm^{-2} min^{-1}) (Table 1, P = 0.1). These data were corrected to a skin temperature of 32°C by the method of Thiele [5]. No trends or correlations with respect to sex, gestational age, or birth weight were observed in this study. CDER values of SGA infants were no different from the remaining population.

DISCUSSION

Basically, two factors, eccrine activity and permeability, determine the magnitude of CDER. Within the limits of this methodology the skin barrier to CO_2 penetration in the healthy term newborn appears at least as efficient as in the adult. Increased CO_2 loss with sweating has been demonstrated by many investigators [4,6]. The contribution of minimally active sweat glands to CDER is not well established. Measurement of CDER on two subjects born with no sweat glands resulted in about the same CDER as in normal subjects in a cool environment. Active sweating appears to increase CDER two to three times [4]. In the absence of sweating CDER is regulated by the permeability characteristics of the skin.

An analysis of CDER variations at different environmental temperatures is not possible with the data presently available. No significant differences were observed between newborn and adult CDER (Table 1) at ambient temperature. The relative change in CDER with sweating would also undoubtedly be small.

If one accepts measurement of CDER as a sensitive index of epidermal barrier

Table 1 Comparison of Corrected CDER Values

	Adults	Neonates
n	30	21
$\bar{x}$, nl cm^{-2} min^{-1}	23.1	21.8
SD, nl cm^{-2} min^{-1}	6.8	5.4
	P = 0.1	

n, number of observations; $\bar{x}$, mean; SD, standard deviation.

Corrected to 32°C following Thiele [5].

Source: Ref. 7.

function, then one may extrapolate these results to other polar compounds. For example, one would expect that alcohol would penetrate neonatal skin at a rate similar to adult skin. Prediction of a similar permeability toward nonpolar compounds should be made cautiously.

SUMMARY

Carbon dioxide emission rates were measured in term newborn and adults with an infrared CO_2 analyzer. No significant emission rate difference existed indicating the skin barrier to CO_2 of the newborn is equal to that of the adult.

REFERENCES

1. Shaw LA, Messer AC, Weiss S: Cutaneous respiration in man. Factors affecting the rate of carbon dioxide elimination and oxygen absorption. Am J Physiol 90:107, 1929.
2. Shaw LA, Messer AC: Cutaneous respiration in man. The effect of temperature and of relative humidity upon the rate of carbon dioxide elimination and oxygen absorption. Am J Physiol 95:13, 1930.
3. Frame GW, Strauss WG, Maibach HI: Carbon dioxide emission of the human arm and hand. J Invest Dermatol 59:155, 1972.
4. Thiele FAJ, Kempen LHJ: A micro method for measuring the carbon dioxide release by small skin areas. Br J Dermatol 86:463, 1972.
5. Thiele FAJ: Measurement on the surface of the skin. Doctoral thesis, 1974.
6. Rothman S: *Physiology and Biochemistry of the Skin*. University of Chicago Press, Chicago, 1954, pp 580-583.
7. Cunico RL, Maibach HI, Kahn H, Bloom E: Skin barrier properties in the newborn; transepidermal water loss and carbon dioxide emission rates. Biol Neonate 32:177-182, 1977.

7

Comparative Skin Barrier Function: Oxygen Diffusion Resistance

HANS T. VERSMOLD
University of Munich, Munich, Federal Republic of Germany

JOHN W. SEVERINGHAUS
University of California Medical School, San Francisco, California

Oxygen flux across human skin was described more than 100 years ago by Gerlach [1]. However, only recently have clinicians become interested in the O_2 diffusional properties of skin. In 1963, Hutchinson et al. [2] postulated that the transdermal route could be used to oxygenate asphyxiated newborns. In this decade Huch et al. [3] and Eberhard et al. [4] demonstrated that a heated O_2 electrode tracks arterial oxygen tension when placed on the skin surface of newborns.

Maturation of human skin implies striking changes of its structure (see Chap. 1) which may affect its properties as a barrier to oxygen diffusion. However, little or nothing is known about maturational changes of related functional properties. There may be a changing blood flow to the skin, a redistribution away from the surface, a changing resistance to oxygen diffusion, and/or a changing oxygen consumption by the skin.

Using two experimental approaches we tried to investigate some of the variables involved. We first examined the P_{O_2} at newborns' unheated skin surface [5], which we found to be closely related to skin blood flow. We also directly measured the resistance of skin to oxygen diffusion [6].

OXYGEN TENSION AT THE UNHEATED SKIN SURFACE

We studied 19 newborns within the first 2 days of life. Their birth weights ranged from 800 to 4100 g, their gestational ages from 24 to 42 weeks. The

PO$_2$ was measured at the skin surface by an unheated Huch [3] PO$_2$ electrode. The infants' arterial PO$_2$ was estimated by a conventional transcutaneous PO$_2$ monitor (TCM 1, Radiometer, Copenhagen).

The PO$_2$ at the unheated skin surface decreased with increasing maturity. In normoxemic infants weighing less than 1500 g the mean PO$_2$ was 27.2 torr, in infants of 1500-2500 g 14.3 torr, and in infants weighing more than 2500 g, 2.9 torr. Skin temperatures were not different in these groups.

The low skin-surface PO$_2$ in the most mature infants did not increase when arterial PO$_2$ was raised by oxygen breathing. However, in the most immature infants skin surface PO$_2$ rose markedly with increasing PaO$_2$ (Fig. 1 [5]). Interestingly, the same pattern of a decreasing skin-surface PO$_2$ with increasing maturity could be observed when babies were born prematurely and lived extra utero. With postnatal maturation their high skin-surface PO$_2$ declined towards a PO$_2$ usually seen in newborns at term. Thus, skin maturation, rather than environmental factors, appears to be responsible for the observed developmental changes in skin-surface PO$_2$.

There is indirect evidence that the PO$_2$ at the unheated skin surface is mainly related to skin blood flow. In four premature infants with moderate hypotension and poor peripheral perfusion skin surface PO$_2$ was relatively low, and rose into the expected range after blood transfusion had normalized their blood pres-

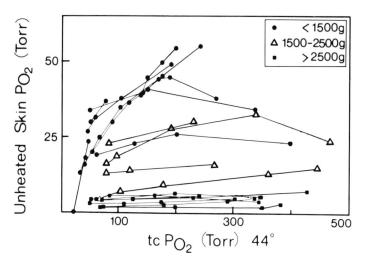

Figure 1   Response of skin surface PO$_2$ to increasing PaO$_2$ (tcPO$_2$ 44°) in 19 newborns. Lines connect PO$_2$ values of each infant at increasing inspiratory oxygen concentrations. (From Ref. 5.)

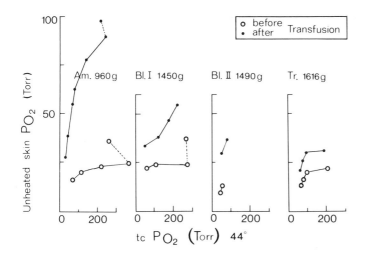

Figure 2 Response of skin surface P$_{O_2}$ to increasing Pa$_{O_2}$ (tcP$_{O_2}$ 44°) in four premature infants before and after blood transfusion. Baby Am received phototherapy during the posttransfusion study. (From Ref. 5.)

sures. (Fig. 2 [5].) Phototherapy, increasing skin blood flow without altering skin temperature, markedly increased skin surface P$_{O_2}$. Crying and/or activity, enhancing peripheral perfusion, greatly increased skin surface P$_{O_2}$, independently of Pa$_{O_2}$.

These observations point to the prevailing importance of skin blood flow in determining the skin-surface P$_{O_2}$. We conclude that the high skin-surface P$_{O_2}$ in premature infants reflects blood flow to their skin in excess of skin oxygen consumption, presumably due to immature control of cutaneous circulation.

RESISTANCE OF SKIN TO OXYGEN DIFFUSION

In addition to high skin blood flow in premature babies, a low resistance of their skin to oxygen diffusion could contribute to the high P$_{O_2}$ on their skin. To investigate the influence of skin maturation on its resistance to oxygen diffusion, we applied the method described by Severinghaus in Chapter 9 to measure skin O$_2$ diffusion resistance directly.

We studied 15 premature and 24 term newborns. Of these, six and two, respectively, were small for gestational age. Gestational ages ranged from 27 to 41 weeks, birth weights from 1060 to 3800 g. Fourteen older children from 0.3 to 14 y of age, and 10 adults were also studied.

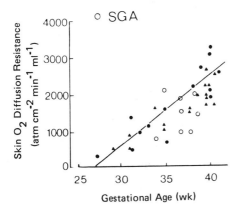

Figure 3 Dependence of skin O_2 diffusion resistance on gestational age in 39 newborns. ○, small-for-gestational-age babies. (Adapted from Ref. 6.)

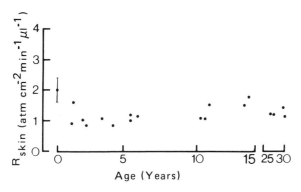

Figure 4 Dependence of skin O_2 diffusion resistance on postnatal age. For term infants the mean ± SD is given.

Skin O_2 diffusion resistance increased linearly with gestational age ($r = 0.87$) or birth weight ($r = 0.81$). This increase was about 10-fold from 27 weeks of gestation to term (Fig. 3). In small-for-gestational-age babies there was a tendency to low resistance values which did not reach the level of significance. From age 1 yr to adulthood skin O_2 diffusion resistance was lower than in newborns at term ($P < 0.05$) (Fig. 4).

In summary, skin maturation is associated with a marked increase in skin O_2

diffusion resistance [6]. This has been confirmed in a repetition of our study (D. Wilson, personal communication). In the mature newborn infant skin O$_2$ diffusion resistance reaches peak values above those in children and adults.

CONCLUSIONS

In premature infants the low O$_2$ diffusion resistance of skin and a high skin blood flow may allow for a high oxygen flux across the skin if there is an appropriate P$_{O_2}$ gradient.

Under normal circumstances no oxygen will be lost from the body across the skin, because the ambient P$_{O_2}$ in air is higher than the mean capillary P$_{O_2}$ in the skin, so that there is an inward P$_{O_2}$ gradient. It had been speculated that oxygen might pass into premature babies through their skin [2]. According to our data this is certainly correct, since the skin of premature babies is virtually no barrier to oxygen diffusion. However, one has to consider that only a small part of total body blood flow passes the skin. Therefore, the amount of transdermal oxygen uptake into the blood must be far too small to allow oxygenation of an hypoxemic premature baby through its skin. This has already been experimentally demonstrated by Avery [7].

On the skin of adults, unlike newborns, transcutaneous P$_{O_2}$ (tcP$_{O_2}$) monitors usually fail to measure tcP$_{O_2}$ values equivalent to arterial P$_{O_2}$. This had been generally attributed to a low O$_2$ permeability of adult skin. According to our data, however, the skin of adults has no higher O$_2$ diffusion resistance than that of newborns. Obviously, the low tcP$_{O_2}$/PaO$_2$ ratio in the adult must be explained by other factors.

ACKNOWLEDGMENT

This work was supported by Deutsche Forschungsgemeinschaft, Grant Ve 32/3.

REFERENCES

1. Gerlach P: Über das Hautathmen. Arch Anat Physiol Lpz 431: 1851.
2. Hutchinson JH, Kerr MM, William KA, Hopkinson WI: Hyperbaric oxygen in the resuscitation of the newborn. Lancet ii:1019, 1963.
3. Huch R, Lübbers EW, Huch A: Quantitative continuous measurement of partial oxygen pressure on the skin of adults and newborn babies. Pflügers Arch Ges Physiol 337:185, 1972.
4. Eberhard P, Hammacher K, Mindt W: Methode zur kutanen Messung des Sauerstoffpartialdruckes. Biomed Technik 18:212, 1972.
5. Versmold HT, Holzmann M, Linderkamp O, Riegel KP: Skin oxygen permeability in premature infants. Pediatrics 62:488, 1978.

6. Versmold HT, Tooley WH, Severinghaus JW: Increase in skin oxygen diffusion resistance with increasing birth weight, in *Continuous Transcutaneous Blood Gas Monitoring*, edited by Huch A, Huch R, Lucey JF. Liss, New York, 1979, pp 271-272.
7. Avery ME: Percutaneous oxygen uptake in infants. Am J Dis Child 100: 565, 1960.

8

Variability in Skin Oxygen Diffusion Resistance Measurement

DONALD R. WILSON, HOWARD MAIBACH, and JOHN W. SEVERINGHAUS
University of California Medical School, San Francisco, California

Great variability exists when measuring O_2 diffusion resistance (R_S). The problem apparently does not extend to the 10 samples of a trial, but lies between trials. The standard errors of trial resistance means are about 10 times greater than the standard errors of resistances within a trial. Some physiological (skin), physical (electrode), technical, or combination variable produces heterogeneous trial mean resistances.

Several possible causes of R_S variability were investigated including comparison of R_S before and after switching electrodes, skin site preparations, temporal resistance fluctuations over a number of days from different skin regions, and temporal fluctuations of a skin region within 24 hr.

METHODS AND RESULTS

Before and After Switching

Rising R_S lowers $P_T O_2$ (Teflon electrode more than $P_M O_2$ (Mylar electrode). Therefore, the value of r (P_T / P_M) would probably be less after switching electrodes if time and measurement affect r.

Existing premature infant, term infant, and adult before and after r means (mean of 10 consecutive measurements) were analyzed with a paired data t-test. Subject r were tested in their respective premature infant, term infant, and adult groupings as well as in a single pooled group. Resistance similarity of the two

Table 1 Mean Before and After Switching Teflon/Mylar Ratios

Group	Mean before ratio	Mean after ratio	Mean ratio	Mean of before-after ratio	Probability
Premature infants	0.665 ±0.051[a]	0.607 ±0.046	+0.059 ±0.041	0.636 ±0.044	0.10 < P < 0.20
Term infants	0.518 ±0.033	0.545 ±0.041	−0.027 ±0.004	0.532 ±0.033	0.30 < P < 0.50
Adults	0.588 ±0.036	0.564 ±0.051	+0.024 ±0.032	0.576 ±0.041	0.30 < P < 0.50
Pooled	0.590 ±0.040	0.572 ±0.046	+0.015 ±0.024	0.581 ±0.039	0.50 < P < 0.70

[a]SE.

adjacent skin sites was tested by comparing P_TO_2 and P_MO_2 values with chi-square.

Table 1 lists the results of the paired data t-tests examining possible reduction of R_S with the second measurement.

No significant changes were found; premature infants demonstrate a questionable insignificant trend towards an initial measurement effect.

A consistent R_S difference between the adjacent skin sites measured with Teflon and Mylar electrodes was tested indirectly with chi-square. The direction of change in the P_TO_2 and P_MO_2 between initial and remeasurement was noted for 29 infant and adult subjects. A P_O_2 increase scored +, a decrease scored -, and no change (initial and remeasurement P_O_2 within 2 mmHg) scored 0. Table 2 presents the matrix of nine possible chi-square categories. The expected probability for each category associated with the hypothesis of no difference between them is 0.111. The categories were grouped into three categories according to the following criteria:

A. ++,00,-- P_TO_2 and P_MO_2 changed in the same direction, possibly responding to fluctuating arterial P_O_2 or time-dependent vasodilation.

B. -+,+-   As Teflon increased, Mylar decreased (or vice versa) upon switching due to a constant skin site R_S difference.

C. 0+,0-,-0,+0   Either Teflon or Mylar changed but the other did not, possibly due to poor electrode preparation or attachment to a skin site.

The distribution of actual and expected scores for each category, calculated chi-square, degrees of freedom, and associated probability are shown in Table 3. Category A contains greater than the expected number of scores; suggesting an insignificant parallel trend ($0.05 < P < 0.10$) of P_TO_2 and P_MO_2. The actual and expected scores indicating an R_S difference between sites were quite similar ($6 \sim 6.44$), failing to show a change from first to second measurement.

Table 2 Initial-Remeasurement P_O_2: Directional Difference Chi-Square Categories

		Mylar		
		+	0	−
	+	++	+0	+−
Teflon	0	0+	00	0−
	−	−+	−0	−−

Table 3 Before-After Switching $P_{T}O_2 - P_{M}O_2$ Trends: Chi-Square

Category	Actual scores	Expected scores	Chi-square	Degrees freedom	Probability
A	15	9.67			
B	6	6.44	4.83	2	$0.05 < P < 0.10$
C	8	12.89			

Skin Site Preparation with Distilled Water, Alcohol, Acetone, and Tape Stripping

The forearm skin of an adult male subject was prepared with distilled water, 70% isopropyl alcohol, acetone, and plastic tape stripping to determine which method best reduced resistance variability. The liquid compounds were applied to a tissue and wiped lightly across the skin site four times. Stripping involved sequentially applying six 15-cm-long sections of Scotch plastic mending tape firmly to the skin site and rapidly pulling them free, removing what adhered to the tape. Each preparation method was tested five times in random sequence with the other preparation trials. Three to four preparations were measured in any 24-hr period; both right and left forearms were employed. The electrodes were prepared and applied to the skin sites as in the infant-adult study and were not switched; only a single set of 10 measurements was taken.

R_S was lowest after stripping, intermediate with acetone, and highest with water and alcohol (Table 4) but the differences were not significant.

Eight R_S Measurements Over 19 Days from Four Skin Sites

R_S was measured on the same skin sites eight times over a 19-day period from the left forearm, left foreleg, left abdomen, and forehead of a single adult male. Preparation and application of the Teflon and Mylar electrodes followed that of the infant-adult R_S study. Electrodes were not switched; a single set of 10 simultaneous $P_{T}O_2$ and $P_{M}O_2$ was recorded.

The trial mean O_2 R_S of the forearm, foreleg, abdomen, and forehead were tested with a simple F test determining regional differences between skin sites. The regions were also compared in groups of two (all combinations) with an unpaired data t-test clarifying where differences probably occur. The results are presented in Table 5; regional R_S means, standard error of the mean, F-test probability, and t-test probability matrix of two region comparisons are shown.

The overall F test probability (0.014) indicates the possible existence of at least one skin region with significantly different ($P < 0.05$) R_S. The t-test prob-

Table 4 Distilled Water, Alcohol, Acetone, and Stripped Skin Preparation
Comparison

Mean and standard error R_S (atm cm^{-2} min^{-1} nl^{-1})

Trials:	Distilled water	Alcohol	Acetone	Stripped skin	Probability
$\overline{X}$	0.001418	0.001673	0.001138	0.000870	
SE	±0.000163	±0.000353	±0.000140	±0.000157	0.099

t-Test probabilities

	Distilled water	Alcohol	Acetone
Alcohol	0.531		
Acetone	0.228	0.196	
Stripped skin	0.042	0.071	0.237

$\overline{X}$, mean; SE, standard error.

Table 5 Forearm, Foreleg, Abdomen, and Forehead R_S

Mean and standard error R_S (atm cm^{-2} min^{-1} nl^{-1})

	Forearm	Foreleg	Abdomen	Forehead	Probability
$\overline{X}$	0.001800	0.001551	0.001618	0.000925	
SE	±0.000232	±0.000146	±0.000140	±0.000183	0.014

t-Test probabilities

	Forearm	Foreleg	Abdomen
Foreleg	0.377		
Abdomen	0.550	0.750	
Forehead	0.011	0.015	0.011

$\overline{X}$, mean; SE, standard error.

ability matrix shows the forehead R_S significantly lower than the other three
sites (P = 0.011, 0.015, and 0.011 with forearm, foreleg, and abdomen, respectively). The forearm, foreleg, and abdomen show strong similarity.

The skin region measurements were taken over a period of days; the presence
of a variable (perhaps physiological) fluctuating with the sampling period and affecting all sites similarly was tested with Kendall coefficient of concordance.

Table 6 Common Fluctuating Daily Variable Tested with Kendall Coefficient of Concordance (w)

	24 May	29 May	1 June	6 June	7 June	12 June
Forearm	3	5	1	6	2	4
Foreleg	1	3	4	2	6	5
Abdomen	2	4	3	5	6	1
Forehead	4	3	2	6	5	1
$\overline{X}$	10	19	10	11	15	19

$\overline{X}$, mean; w = 280; sum of squares = 92; P > 0.05.

With s = 92 < 143.3 (P = 0.05), no significant common variable affecting all regions similarly appears to exist.

The mean daily R_S measurements of each skin site were ranked and compared; the result is presented in Table 6.

Forearm R_S Measured Within 24 hr

R_S was measured from three left and three right forearm sites of one man within 24 hr to determine if resistance variability was as great as when sampling the same site over several days. Decreased variability for the 24-hr period would suggest a slowly changing physiological variable effective on resistances taken days apart.

The six forearm R_S trials obtained in 24 hr were tested with a simple F test for significant variability; trials in groups of two (all combinations) were tested with an unpaired data t-test to help locate areas of significant difference (Table 7). The mean and standard error of the mean R_S of all trials are shown along with a matrix of t-test probabilities from the unpaired data t-comparisons.

Since the F test produced an associated probability (< 0.000000) < 0.01, highly significant variability is apparent within the six forearm measurements. The t-test matrix shows all group comparisons producing highly significant differences between trials ($P < 0.01$) except trials 2 versus 3 ($P = 0.147$); significant variability between trials appears widespread.

The forearm R_S obtained within 24 hr were compared with those taken over a number of days (section c) by testing the respective trial means with an unpaired data t-test (Table 8).

Since t = 0.571 with 12 degrees of freedom associates with P = 0.590, no significant differences ($P > 0.05$) appear between the 24 hr and number of days

Table 8 Forearm R_S in 24 hr

Mean and standard error R_S ($atm\ cm^{-2}\ min^{-1}\ nl^{-1}$)

	Right arm trials			Left arm trials			Probability
	1	2	3	4	5	6	
$\overline{X}$	0.001939	0.002131	0.002059	0.002309	0.001565	0.001752	< 0.000000
SE (±)	0.000036	0.000044	0.000016	0.000022	0.000012	0.000023	

t-Test probabilities

		Trials			
	1	2	3	4	5
2	0.003303				
3	0.006746	0.147106			
Trials 4	0.000000	0.001843	0.000000		
5	0.000000	0.000000	0.000000	0.000000	
6	0.000355	0.000000	0.000000	0.000000	0.000001

$\overline{X}$, mean; SE, standard error.

Table 8 Forearm R_S, 24 hr Sample Versus Days

	Mean	Standard error	t	Degrees of freedom	Probability
24 hr	0.001959	0.001110	0.571	12	0.590
Days	0.001800	0.000232			

Table 9 Right Versus Left Forearm R_S (atm cm^{-2} min^{-1} nl^{-1})

	Mean	Standard error	t	Degrees of freedom	Probability
Right	0.002043	±0.000024	2.49	58	0.012
Left	0.001875	±0.000060			

Since t = 2.49 associates with P = 0.012, a small but significant (P < 0.05) difference appears to exist between forearms.

samples. Inspection of the respective standard errors, however, reveals that 24-hr sample variability is half that of the measurements taken over a number of days.

The three right and three left forearm trials were respectively pooled and tested with an unpaired data t-test detecting any difference between forearms (Table 9); right R_S appears greater.

DISCUSSION

The variability observed between the previous infant and adult subjects may be more than normal subject variation deriving instead from within-subject variation. Such variability was presently discovered for a single subject and contained approximately the same degree of variability as between-subjects. Assuming other subjects will produce similar individual variability, that between-subjects may be reduced by sampling an individual several times, and taking means for analysis, the mean extremes should be less than that of actual R_S. Repetitive individual measurement, however, beyond two or three trials (10 samples per trial) is time-consuming, inconvenient to the subject, and generally impractical, thereby necessitating an actual solution to the variability problem.

The variation apparently does not originate from remeasurement of sites following electrode switching, particularly in term infants and adults (premature infants may be affected, Table 1); a consistent R_S difference between the two adjacent electrode sites also seems an improbable source since A and not B was inflated (Table 3).

The distilled water, alcohol, acetone, and skin stripping forearm preparations all failed to reduce between-trial variability to an insignificant level (all F test $P < 0.000000$); however, visual inspection of the preparation standard errors in Table 4 reveals that acetone produced the least amount of between-trial variation.

The stripped skin R_S tend, insignificantly (Table 4), to be lower than the other preparations possibly because stripping reduces stratum corneum thickness (hence, layers of resistance) through partial removal of outer cells. The large variability observed between all respective preparation trials possibly masked detection. A small sample size increase may be needed to detect a significant stripping effect.

The forearm, foreleg, abdomen, and forehead region study (Table 5) demonstrated that: (1) all regions generated appreciable variability and (2) forehead R_S appeared significantly lower than the other three regions. The forearm and abdomen resistances overlap considerably and support the assumption that adult forearm and infant abdomen resistance can be compared without significant effect from skin region variation. This study also demonstrated the improbable existence of an R_S variable slowly fluctuating over several days but affecting all skin regions identically.

The forearm R_S trials obtained in 24 hr demonstrated highly significant between-trial variability (Table 7); however, visual comparison of the standard errors of the 24 hr and period of days samples (Table 8) shows that the former produced half as much variability. Significant resistance difference apparently exists between right and left forearms, but is small.

We believe that preparing the skin site with acetone, taking repetitive R_S measurement trials closely in time and averaging, and perhaps recording from homologous regions on all subjects may help reduce resistance variability between subjects. The major cause of variability, whether physiological, physical, or technical, remains undefined and unsolved.

SUMMARY

R_S variability in term newborns and adults was investigated analyzing R_S before and after switching electrodes, various skin site preparations, temporal R_S fluctuations over a number of days from different skin regions, and temporal R_S fluctuation of a single region over 24 hr. The following conclusions were reached:

1. Variation does not apparently originate from remeasurement of sites following electrode switching.
2. Distilled water, alcohol, acetone, and skin-stripping forearm preparations all

failed to remove significant variability between trials; acetone produced relatively less variability.

3. Forearm, foreleg, abdomen, and forehead all generated appreciable variability; forehead R_S appeared significantly lower than the others.
4. Forearm and abdomen R_S appear comparable.
5. Forearm R_S measurement in one subject over 24 hr and several days both produced significant between-trial variability; the 24-hr measurements, however, produced half as much variability.
6. Right forearm R_S appeared slightly greater than the left.
7. The major cause of variability remains undefined and unsolved; a small reduction in variability may result by preparing the site with acetone, taking repetitive R_S measurement trials close in time and averaging, and measuring from homologous regions.

9

Resistance of Skin to Oxygen Diffusion

JOHN W. SEVERINGHAUS

University of California Medical School, San Francisco, California

Oxygen diffusional resistance, or conductance, may be determined by using a skin-surface oxygen electrode. Transcutaneous measurement of PO_2 has been established during the last decade by Huch et al. in Marburg, and by Eberhard in Basel. A polarographic electrode is self-heated to 43-45°C and placed on skin surface. The resulting vasodilation under the electrode increases skin superficial blood flow to about 0.5 ml blood per gram of skin per minute, which is about 10-50 times more than needed to supply the skin's metabolic needs for O_2. As a result, surface PO_2 rises to about equal the arterial PO_2, P_aO_2.

Transcutaneous PO_2 electrodes based on this principle are now in use primarily in newborn nurseries to monitor continuously the PO_2 in infants who need O_2 supplementation, and are thus at risk of developing retrolentil fibroplasia. Both PO_2 and PCO_2 electrodes may be mounted on the chest. The mounting ring is attached to skin with doublesided adhesive tape, with a drop of water or other gel between the electrode surface and the skin to exclude air. The skin under the electrode is heated to the point of a first degree burn, and remains reddened for 6-24 hr after removal of the electrode.

In Figure 1, the recording illustrates several periods of apnea due to upper airway obstruction.

A polarographic O_2 electrode consumes O_2, and measures the resulting current. A platinum or gold cathode, polarized about -0.7 v versus silver, is covered with a membrane of plastic with limited permeability to O_2. By choosing the appropriate membrane and cathode diameter, it is possible to obtain a current

131

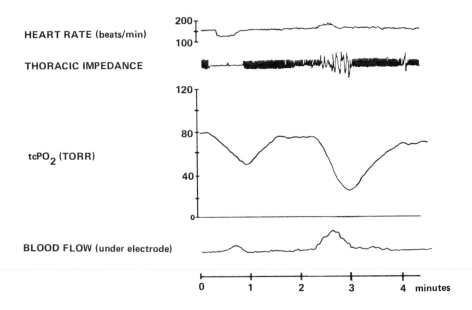

Figure 1 Two episodes of obstructive apnea in a premature infant, showing the resulting rapid fall in tcPO$_2$. The impedance trace shows increased respiratory effort during the second apnea, indicative of obstruction. (Courtesy of Dr. Joyce Peabody, Children's Hospital, San Francisco, California.)

which is a linear function of the PO$_2$ outside the membrane, and to keep the O$_2$ consumption so low that about 95% of the O$_2$ gradient is within the membrane even when O$_2$ must flow through skin first to reach the electrode.

Figure 2 illustrates the geometry of a tcPO$_2$ electrode mounted on skin, and the theoretic distribution of temperature and PO$_2$. The electrode heats the skin and its capillaries to within 2° of the electrode temperature. Thus, inflowing blood undergoes heating, which elevates the blood PO$_2$ about 6% °C if saturation is incomplete, and about 6 torr °C at PO$_2$ levels above 100 torr. Skin metabolism uses some O$_2$, reducing PO$_2$ in the capillary by about 20 torr, and tissue PO$_2$ falls about another 30 torr between the capillary and the surface. The heat-induced rise and the metabolism-induced fall approximately cancel so that surface PO$_2$ may simulate P$_a$O$_2$.

Since the tcPO$_2$ electrode consumes O$_2$, it may be used to measure the resistance of skin to the diffusion of O$_2$ under special conditions [1]. The Roche tcPO$_2$ electrode has a 4-mm diameter gold cathode which is ideal for this purpose. To measure resistance, the mylar membrane usually employed on this

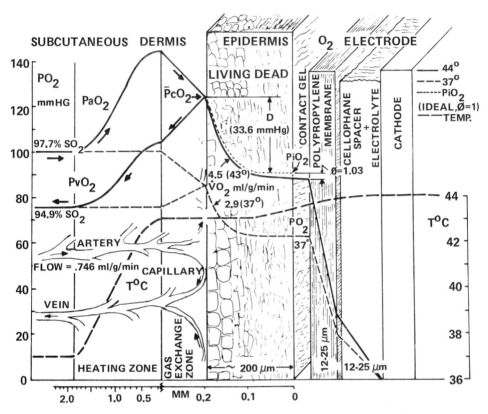

Figure 2 Schema of the profiles of temperature and P_{O_2} within the skin and electrode membranes, based on data obtained in nine normal adults. The dashed P_{O_2} line would be found with a non-O_2-consuming electrode. (From Ref. 2.)

electrode is replaced by Teflon, which is about 250 times more permeable to O_2. The electrode then consumes O_2 faster than it can diffuse out through skin, and the fall of skin surface P_{O_2} that results from the measured O_2 flux can be measured. The technique is shown schematically as an electric analog in Figure 3. The two resistances, skin and membrane, are shown in series between the source capillaries, and the sink or ground, at the cathode inside the electrode. The O_2 molecules which reach the cathode react to become OH^-, which means that P_{O_2} is zero at the surface. The effective resistance of the membrane and electrode are measured by observing the current in air or gas of known P_{O_2}. The large cathode permits easy calculation of the area of diffusion. The electrical equiva-

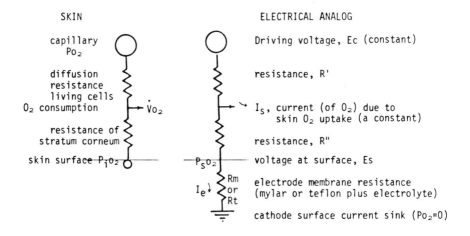

Without an electrode consuming O_2, but with surface occluded, skin surface Po_2 is ideal P_io_2, lower than capillary P_co_2 due to $I_s \times R'$. With electrode on surface (right schema), P_so_2 falls below P_io_2 due to I_e. Electrode measures I_e, but is calibrated in gas to read $Po_2 = P_so_2$, thus defining Rm or Rt.

Mylar: $P_s^m o_2/P_i o_2 = Rm/(R'+R''+Rm)$

Teflon: $P_s^t o_2/P_i o_2 = Rt/(R'+R''+Rt)$

Solve simultaneously for $(R'+R'')$ and $P_i o_2$.

Figure 3 Electrical analog of the skin resistance measurement method. Since PO_2 can be measured with two widely different known membrane resistances, skin resistance can be calculated from Ohm's law.

lent of O_2, computed from Faraday's constant, is 3.48 ml O_2 min^{-1} amp^{-1}. The effective resistance of Teflon (25 μm thick) and Mylar (6 μm with this electrode (including a small correction for edge diffusion, and for the resistance of the thin film of electrolyte within the electrode), were 1.39 and 32.1 atm cm^{-2} min^{-1} μl^{-1}, respectively.

In practice, two measurements are taken, one with Mylar and one with Teflon membrane. Assuming the capillary PO_2 to be constant, and unaffected by the O_2 consumption of the electrode, one writes two equations for the PO_2 drop across series resistors, using Ohm's law, and solves them simultaneously. The result not only gives skin resistance but also "ideal" skin PO_2: the value which would be determined by an electrode which had no O_2 consumption.

We have also found it possible to use the tcPO_2 electrodes to measure skin

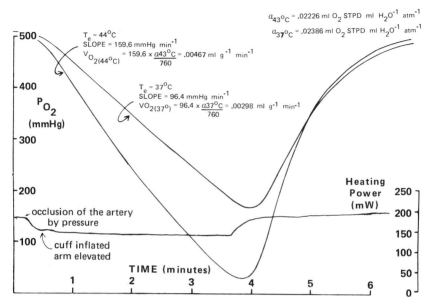

Figure 4 Fall of tcPo$_2$ under two electrodes, one at 37°C, the other at 44°C, when arterial circulation is blocked with an upper arm tourniquet in an adult breathing 100% O$_2$. The linear portion of the falling Po$_2$ is used to compute skin O$_2$ consumption, and the initial Po$_2$ is used to estimate blood flow (with other corrections). (From Ref. 2.)

O$_2$ consumption and blood flow [2]. Figure 4 illustrates the fall of PO$_2$ on skin when blood flow is abruptly stopped by a toruniquet on the upper arm above the electrode. The subject was breathing O$_2$, and tcPo$_2$ was 500 torr. The linear fall occurs as skin uses the dissolved O$_2$. Since solubility is known, O$_2$ consumption can be measured. Flow can be calculated from the initial tcPo$_2$, together with measurement of P$_a$O$_2$, since the O$_2$ consumption is entirely supplied from the dissolved O$_2$ in the passing blood. Small corrections are made for the diffusion gradient within the skin, which is measured at low Po$_2$. Figure 4 also indicates the temperature coefficient of skin metabolism, the Po$_2$ falling faster at 44°C.

Versmold in Munich and Wilson in San Francisco have used these methods to study the relationship of gestational age and weight to skin O$_2$ diffusional resistance. Their separate studies, which follow, are in good agreement with each other and with the adults studied by Eberhard and me [1].

REFERENCES

1. Eberhard P, Severinghaus JW: Measurement of heated skin O_2 diffusion, conductance and Po_2 sensor induced gradients. Acta Anaesthesiol Scand [Suppl] 68:1-3, 1978.
2. Thunstrom AM, Stafford MJ, Severinghaus JW: A two temperature two Po_2 method of estimating the determinants of $tcPO_2$. In *Continuous Transcutaneous Blood Gas Monitoring*, edited by Huch A, Huch R, Lucey JF. Alan R. Liss, New York, for the National Foundation-March of Dimes, BD:OAS XV(4): 167-182, 1979.

10

Comparative Percutaneous Absorption

RONALD C. WESTER and HOWARD MAIBACH
University of California Medical School, San Francisco, California

Little is known about percuraneous absorption in the infant. Yet, it is in the infant where the greatest toxicological response has been seen following topical administration. This chapter deals with parameters of percutaneous absorption, some of the features unique to infants which make them susceptible to toxicity from topical administration, and some unique absorption pharmacokinetics in the infant. This new area of concern demands attention.

SKIN BARRIER DEVELOPMENT AND PERCUTANEOUS ABSORPTION IN PREMATURE AND FULL-TERM INFANTS

The main factor governing percutaneous absorption is the permeability barrier of skin. One major barrier resides principally in the stratum corneum. The critical factor in protection of the infant from the environment is whether the barriers are intact. Intact barriers provide the infant some protection. If the barriers are not intact, any foreign substance coming in contact with the skin may readily be absorbed into the body.

In animal studies (rat, guinea pig) the development of the stratum corneum was observed through fetal life [1]. The genesis of the permeability barrier starts in the last quarter of gestation and is concluded just before term. At birth, the ultrastructure of the stratum corneum is indistinguishable from that of the adult. We do not know when barrier function is completed in the human infant. However, a normal full-term infant probably has a fully developed stratum corneum and intact barrier function [2].

The preterm infant does not have intact barrier function. Nachman and Esterly [3] suggest that preterm infants have increased skin permeability. Skin permeability in preterm infants was evaluated by observing the blanching response to topically applied Neo-Synephrine. Infants 28-34 weeks of gestational age had a rapid response; infants 35-37 weeks responded less dramatically, and infants 38-42 weeks in most instances failed to respond. This is indirect evidence of skin permeability, however it is consistent with the animal data. Preterm infants probably do not have intact barrier function and would show enhanced skin permeability.

If preterm infants are susceptible to enhanced skin penetration, then they would also be more susceptible to systemic toxicity from a topically applied compound. Greaves and co-workers [4] determined the concentration of hexachlorophene in serial blood samples taken from seven premature infants washed with pHisoHex. Systemic absorption was detected at 4 hr. Peak blood levels occurred between days 2 and 4 after a single application on the first day of life. Peak blood levels of hexachlorophene were in the range of 0.75-1.37 $\mu g/ml$. These levels were considerably higher than those observed in full-term infants who had undergone the same washing procedure. They concluded that the dermal absorption of hexachlorophene was greater in premature than in full-term infants. If this is true for hexachlorophene, then it might be true for any potentially toxic material applied to the skin of premature infants.

One further important point concerning skin development is the corresponding development of the metabolizing potential of skin. It is not known what role skin metabolism might play in skin permeability or whether skin metabolism might detoxify a potentially dangerous substance as it is absorbed. In animals the development of the metabolism potential seems to occur concurrent with the final stage in the development of the stratum corneum [1]. The preterm infant might lack the skin metabolizing potential of the full-term infant. This requires experimental evaluation.

Other studies document the functional capability of the neonate skin compared to the adult. The stratum corneum functions examined are transepidermal water loss, oxygen transport, carbon dioxide transport, and chloride flux. Details are in Chapters 5-10. In general the ability of the stratum corneum to contain these moieties appears well-developed in the neonate.

FACTORS AFFECTING PERCUTANEOUS ABSORPTION

Dose Concentration and Surface Area

When a compound comes in contact with skin the amount of absorption will depend on many factors. Foremost among these are concentration of applied dose and surface area. As the concentration of applied dose increases, the efficiency of absorption (percentage) can change. However, a more relevant point is that as the applied dose is increased the total amount absorbed into the body increases [5,6]. Increasing applied dose, therefore, increases the potential for toxicity. The other parameter closely associated with dose is surface area. Increasing the surface are of applied dose increases the absorption [7]. Therefore, the greatest potential for percutaneous absorption can occur when a high concentration of compound is spread over a large part of the body.

Skin Site of Application

Regional variation in absorption occurs depending on which anatomical site the compound is applied. This is true for humans [8,9] and animals [10]. In humans the anatomic site of greatest absorption is the scrotum where most of the applied compound is absorbed [8]. Other anatomic sites of high absorption are the scalp, forehead, and postauricular region. Therefore, the potential for systemic toxicity is increased for those anatomic sites where enhanced absorption occurs. A related point is that there is regional variation in primary skin irritation for human and animal [11] skin. That the potential for skin irritation is related to the potential for skin absorption has not been shown; however, such a possibility appears plausible.

Occlusion

Percutaneous absorption is increased if the site of application is occluded. Occlusion is a covering of the applied dose, either intentional as with bandaging or unintentional, such as putting on clothing (diaper, rubber pants) after applying a topical compound. Occlusion is a combination of many physical factors affecting skin and the applied compound. Occlusion changes the hydration and temperature of the skin, which affect absorption. Occlusion also prevents the accidental wiping off or evaporation (volatile compound) of the applied compound, in essence maintaining a higher applied dose.

Skin Condition

Skin conditions other than hydration and temperature affect percutaneous absorption. The most obvious is loss of barrier function of the stratum corneum through disease or damage. Absorption can be virtually 100% if all barrier function is removed. However, removing one major barrier, the stratum corneum, does not lead to complete loss of barrier function. In adults, stripping the stratum corneum with cellophane tape produces less penetration enhancement of hydrocortisone than does occlusion [12]. Virtually any type of change in skin condition, especially change in the barrier function of the stratum corneum, whether natural or inflicted, will change the percutaneous absorption of the skin.

Vehicle

A. H. Beckett noted that "a drug is not given to man: what is given is a preparation containing the drug." This is true for topical vehicles because they both influence the percutaneous absorption of the drug and exert their own effect on the skin. Percutaneous absorption of a drug from a vehicle depends in part on the partition of the drug between the vehicle and the skin. In addition to drug solubility, factors such as drug concentration and pH can influence the interaction between vehicle, drug, and skin. The vehicle can change the integrity of the skin and this will influence absorption. An example would be an occlusive vehicle which would alter skin hydration. Vehicles can contain an agent such as urea which will enhance percutaneous absorption, or the vehicle itself will enhance absorption. The best example of the latter is dimethylsulfoxide (DMSO) which readily permeates skin and by "solvent drag" causes enhanced penetration. Thus, the vehicle is so important that its influence on absorption should not be minimized in an absorption study.

Multiple Dose Application

Percutaneous absorption studies are usually conducted using a single application. By some analytical means the amount absorbed is determined and the percentage of absorption of that compound is calculated. This is fine for the limits of the study, but the question remains as to its relevance to the clinical situation. A topically administered compound (prescribed or exposed contamination) can be applied more frequently than once a day, and the topical exposure can be chronic. This is a new area in the pharmacokinetics of skin absorption. Initial studies show a difference in skin absorption with repetitive daily application and with daily chronic application. Absorption from one application of a high concentration (hydrocortisone, testosterone) was greater than when the same concentration was applied in divided doses [10,13]. The absorption of hydrocortisone significantly increased during chronic administration. Absorption from day 8 application was 144-275% greater than from day 1 application [14]. Similarly, with chronic administration of salicyclic acid, the penetration flux increased during the first 5 days of application. Penetration flux then decreased with weekly application [15]. In both of these studies involving chronic application the authors suggest that the initial applications of compound altered the condition of the stratum corneum and this altered barrier function resulted in the different absorption for subsequent applications.

Metabolism

One method the body uses to protect itself is the metabolism of foreign bodies and drugs. The organ most associated with metabolism is the liver. Any ingested substance as it is absorbed from the gastrointestinal tract must first pass through the liver. Here any potentially toxic material can be biotransformed into inactive metabolites. Other "first contact" organs, the lung and skin, also are capable of metabolizing drugs and foreign substances. The skin contains most of the functionalization reactions of liver; the phase I oxidative, reductive, and hydrolytic reactions; and the phase II conjugation reactions. The metabolizing potential of skin has been estimated to be about 2% of that of the liver [16].

The skin, by possessing most of the functionalizing reactions of metabolism, is also capable of transforming nontoxic foreign substances into toxic materials. An example of this is benzo[a]pyrene, an ingredient of tar and pollutants. Benzo[a]pyrene itself is not carcinogenic. However, the diolepoxides of benzo-[a]pyrene which bind to nucleic acids are formed in skin and are carcinogenic [16].

INFANTILE POISONING BY TOPICAL APPLICATION

Lundell and Nordman [17] reported the case of a 2-week-old infant who developed reddish, patchy eczema in the inguinal regions, on the upper part of the thighs, and axilla. Part of the treatment was to paint the areas with Castellani's solution, an antimicrobial containing phenol and resorcinol. The infant became cyanotic and was in critical condition for days.

Infected skin had damaged barrier function so there was little resistance to absorption. Additionally, the inguinal region and the axilla are sites of enhanced absorption [8]. The situation was further jeopardized in that by painting on the Castellani's solution, the dose was spread over a large surface area; this enhanced the potential for increased systemic availability [7].

Brown [18] and Armstrong and co-workers [19] reported separate cases of phenolic disinfectants in the hospital laundry causing death of infants and sickening others. By having the toxic compounds in clothing such as diapers, the compounds were spread over a large surface area on a skin site with enhanced absorption. Both parameters (large surface area and application to the urorectal area) enhance absorption [8-10]. If the diaper was covered with rubber pants or more clothing, this would also enhance absorption and the potential for systemic availability.

Feinblatt and co-workers [20] reported the case of a male infant born after 36 weeks of gestation who was treated for bullous lesions with 0.25% hydrocortisone. The child developed cushingoid features and edema which cleared only when hydrocortisone treatment was discontinued. It was subsequently learned that at least 120 g of lotion containing a total of 300 mg of hydrocortisone had been applied to the skin over 8-9 days.

The infant was probably borderline preterm and its barrier function may not have been intact. This could have resulted in enhanced skin absorption. Percutaneous absorption of hydrocortisone increased with chronic administration [14]. Finally, clothing over the site of application might have occluded it and led to further enhanced penetration.

For about 20 years the toxic potential of topically applied hexachlorophene was not recognized. In France in 1972 there was a hexachlorophene-related baby disaster. This involved about 40 deaths from the use of baby powder accidentally contaminated with 6.6% hexachlorophene. The powder normally contains no hexachlorophene. Brain damage occurs in animals when the use of hexachlorophene. Brain damage occurs in animals when the use of hexachlorophene produces whole blood levels around 1 μg/ml. Studies on newborn babies washed (and rinsed off) for 3-5 days with a 3% hexachlorophene-containing antibacterial sudsing emulsion revealed blood levels dangerously close to this (up to 0.8 μg/ml). This provides a small margin of safety especially if babies were exposed continuously to this procedure by conscientious mothers [21].

The above clinical cases illustrate that, either through error or misjudgment, potentially toxic materials can be applied to infant skin. The parameters which govern skin absorption can have an enhancing effect on skin penetration. The results can be fatal (Table 1).

PERCUTANEOUS ABSORPTION IN THE NEWBORN AND SYSTEMIC AVAILABILITY

A study was done to assess the percutaneous absorption in the newborn rhesus monkey [22] (Table 2). Skin absorption in the rhesus monkey is similar in many respects to humans [23-26]. The study showed that absorption in the full-term newborn was the same as the adult (Figure 1).

With one other newborn rhesus, a topical dose of 40 μg/cm^2 was applied to the ventral forearm and the area was occluded with Saran wrap and adhesive tape for 24 hr. Percutaneous absorption was 14.7%, a value twice that from nonoccluded absorption.

The study showed that a high percentage of a steroid can be absorbed through the skin of an infant. The study also suggested an interesting relationship between the skin surface area of a newborn and the system availability of the applied compound.

Once the compound (and/or metabolites) is absorbed, it is available systemically. In the newborn the ratio of surface area (square centimeters) to body weight (kilograms) is three times that of the adult. Therefore, given equal application

Table 1 Infantile Poisoning

Incidence of skin contact	Clinical indications	Possible skin absorption factor involved
Eczema (inguinal region, thigh, axilla) treated with Castellani's solution [17]	Cyanotic	Damaged skin has high absorption; application sites have high absorption; large surface area contact
Phenolic disinfectants in hospital laundry [18,19]	Death	Large surface area contact; clothing may have occlusive effect; urorectal area has high absorption
Bullous lesions treated with hydro-cortisone [20]	Cushingoid	Possible borderline preterm; damaged skin has high absorption; total chronic dose was large; chronic application of hydrocortisone has enhanced absorption; clothing may have occlusive effect
Hexachlorophene in baby powder [21]	Death	Application to large surface area; high concentration of hexachlorophene (6.6%); clothing may have occlusive effect; chronic application

Table 2 Percutaneous Absorption of Testosterone in Newborn Rhesus Monkey

	% dose absorbed[a]	
Time (hr)	4 μg/cm^2	40 μg/cm^2
0-24	6.3 ± 0.9	1.3 ± 0.4
24-48	8.0 ± 0.7	2.1 ± 0.8
48-72	4.3 ± 0.2	1.6 ± 0.6
72-96	2.5 ± 1.1	1.0 ± 0.1
96-120	1.4 ± 0.4	0.7 ± 0.2
Total	22.5 ± 2.2	6.8 ± 2.1

[a]Mean values and standard deviations of three animals. Topical values were corrected for incomplete urinary excretion with the formula

$$\% \text{ absorbed} = \frac{\% \text{ urinary radioactivity topical}}{\% \text{ urinary radioactivity iv}} \times 100.$$

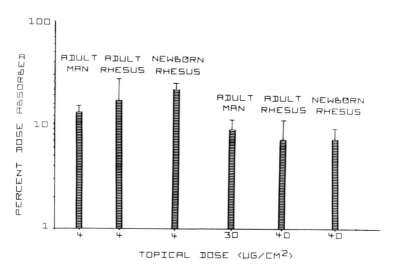

Figure 1 Comparison of percutaneous absorption of testosterone in newborn rhesus, adult rhesus, and adult man. (*Source:* Ref. 22, reproduced with the permission of the International Pediatric Research Foundation, Inc.)

Table 3 Systemic Availability in Newborn and Adult Following Topical Application[a]

	Adult	Infant
Surface area	17,000 cm^2	2200 cm^2 (13% of adult)
Topical dose	100 mg	13 mg (13% of adult)
Patient weight	70 kg	3.4 kg (neonate)
Systemic dose	$\dfrac{100 \text{ mg} \times 0.2 \text{ abs}}{70 \text{ kg}} = 0.28$ mg/kg	$\dfrac{3 \text{ mg} \times 0.2 \text{ abs}}{3.4 \text{ kg}} = 0.76$ mg/kg

[a]Systemic dose = mg/kg; compound = 20% absorbed.

area of skin per newborn and adult, the systemic absorption seen in the newborn can be much more when based on kilograms of body weight (Table 3).

Therefore, by topically applying the same strength compound to both the adult and the newborn, the systemic availability in the newborn is 2.7 times that of the adult. With a different ratio of skin surface to body weight, the therapeutic ratio probably is lower in the newborn than in the adult when the compound is applied topically. This increased systemic availability in the newborn would also be interrelated with any differences in systemic metabolism between the newborn and the adult.

DISCUSSION

This review, like so many others on percutaneous absorption, included a section on the parameters which affect percutaneous absorption. What is most interesting (and in some cases tragic) is that these parameters become extremely important in the newborn. For example, lack of intact barrier function (preterm, disease) can translate into systemic poisoning. Covering a topically applied compound with diaper and rubber pants may act as an occluding device. Occlusion results in enhanced absorption. Other parameters such as chronic dosing and site of application also contribute to enhanced absorption. When some or all of these parameters are involved, absorption from topical administration is enhanced.

The pharmacokinetic parameters which follow absorption (distribution, metabolism, and excretion) are not the subject matter for this review. However, for the sake of completeness, it needs to be mentioned that the infant must deal with the absorbed dose once that becomes systemically available. Any disposition, metabolism, or excretion which was different in the newborn could change the toxic potential of the applied dose.

REFERENCES

1. Singer EJ, Wegmann PC, Lehman, MD, Christensen, MS, Vinson LJ: Barrier development, ultrastructure, and sulfhydryl content of the fetal epidermis. J Soc Cosmet Chem 22:119-137, 1971.
2. Rasmussen JE: Percutaneous absorption in children, in *1979 Year Book of Dermatology*, edited by Dobson RL. Year Book Med. Pub. Inc., Chicago, 1979, pp 25-38.
3. Nachman RL, Esterly NB: Increased skin permeability in preterm infants. J Pediat 79:628-632, 1971.
4. Greaves SJ, Ferry DG, McQueen EG, Malcolm DS, Buckfield PM: Serial hexachlorophene blood levels in the premature infant. N Zealand Med J 81:334-336, 1975.
5. Wester RC, Maibach HI: Relationship of topical dose and percutaneous absorption in rhesus monkey and man. J Invest Dermatol 67:518-520, 1976.
6. Scheuplein RJ, Ross LW: Mechanism of percutaneous absorption. V. Percutaneous absorption of solvent deposited solids. J Invest Dermatol 62:353-360, 1974.
7. Noonan PK, Wester RC: Percutaneous absorption of nitroglycerin. J Pharm Sci 69:365-366, 1980.
8. Feldmann RJ, Maibach HI: Regional variation in percutaneous penetration of ^{14}C cortisone in man. J Invest Dermatol 48:181-183, 1967.
9. Maibach HI, Feldmann RJ, Milby TH, Serat WF: Regional variation in percutaneous penetration in man. Pestic Arch Environ Health 23:208-211, 1971.
10. Wester RC, Noonan PK, Maibach HI: Variations in percutaneous absorption of testosterone in the rhesus monkey due to anatomic site of application and frequency of application. Arch Dermatol Res 267:229-235, 1980.
11. Vinegar MB: Regional variation in primary skin irritation and corrosivity potential in rabbits. Toxicol Appl Pharmacol 49:63-69, 1979.
12. Feldmann R, Maibach HI: Percutaneous penetration of hydrocortisone. II. The effect of stripping and occlusion. Arch Dermatol 91:661-665, 1965.
13. Wester RC, Noonan PK, Maibach HI: Frequency of application on percutaneous absorption of hydrocortisone. Arch Dermatol 113:620-622, 1977.
14. Wester RC, Noonan PK, Maibach HI: Percutaneous absorption of hydrocortisone increases with long-term administration: in vivo studies in the rhesus monkey. Arch Dermatol 116:186-188, 1980.
15. Roberts MS, Horlock E: Effect of repeated skin application on percutaneous absorption of salicyclic acid. J Pharm Sci 67:1685-1687, 1978.
16. Pannatier A, Jenner B, Testa B, Etter JC: The skin as a drug-metabolizing organ. Drug Metab Rev 8:319-343, 1978.
17. Lundell E, Nordman R: A case of infantile poisoning by topical application of Castellani's solution. Ann Clin Res 5:404-406, 1973.
18. Brown BW: Fatal phenol poisoning from improperly laundered diapers. Am J Public Health 60:901-902, 1970.

19. Armstrong RW, Eichner ER, Klein DE, Barthel WF, Bennett JV, Jonsson V, Bruce H, Loveless LE: Pentachlorophenol poisoning in a nursery for newborn infants. II. Epidemiologic and toxicologic studies. J Pediatr 75:317-325 (1969).

20. Feinblatt BI: Aceto T Jr, Beckhorn G, Bruck E: Percutaneous absorption of hydrocortisone in children. Am J Dis Child 112:218-224, 1966.

21. Marzulli FN, Maibach HI: Relevance of animal models: The hexachlorophene story, in *Animal Models in Dermatology*, edited by Maibach HI. Churchill Livingstone, New York, 1975, pp 156-167.

22. Wester RC, Noonan PK, Cole MP, Maibach HI: Percutaneous absorption of testosterone in the newborn rhesus monkey: comparison to the adult. Pediatr Res 11:737-739 (1977).

23. Wester RC, Maibach HI: Percutaneous absorption in the rhesus monkey compared to man. Toxicol Appl Pharmacol 32:394-398, 1975.

24. Wester RC, Maibach HI: Rhesus monkey as an animal model for percutaneous absorption, in *Animal Models in Dermatology*, edited by Maibach HI. Churchill Livingstone, New York, 1975, pp 133-137.

25. Wester RC, Maibach HI: Percutaneous absorption in man and animal: a perspective, in *Cutaneous Toxicity*, edited by Drill V and Lazar P. Academic Press, New York, 1977, pp. 111-126.

26. Wester RC, Noonan PK, Maibach HI: Recent advances in percutaneous absorption using the rhesus monkey model. J Soc Cosmet Chem 30:297-307 (1979).

11

An In Vitro Comparison of the Permeability of Adult Versus Neonatal Skin

JOHN J. McCORMACK, EDWARD K. BOISITS, and L. B. FISHER
Johnson and Johnson Baby Products Company, Skillman, New Jersey

Numerous reports during the last 50 years have documented systemic poisoning in infants after the use of topical products. There have been the relatively recent problems with hexachlorophene poisoning and a variety of corticosteroids, particularly the fluorinated steroids [1-8]. These instances have lead to the assumption that infant skin is more permeable than adult skin. The 31st Meeting of the Over the Counter Miscellaneous External Drug Review Panel issued a monograph stating "Neonatal skin is more permeable than adult skin." What evidence is there to support this?

There is in vivo evidence that the skin of premature infants is more permeable to phenylephrine than mature full-term infants [9]. In contrast, results of additional in vivo experiments suggest that the lower transepidermal water loss of full-term infants as compared to adults indicates an even better barrier [10]. The question examined in this paper is: What are the differences and/or similarities in the penetrability of baby versus adult skin?

The value and limitations of in vitro systems in helping to explain and predict percutaneous absorption in vivo has been examined [11,12]. The specific question we address does not now lend itself to being examined in vivo. There are practical reasons why penetration of a group of substances through the skin of a newborn has not been measured. Therefore, we produced a system and a program designed, within the limits of in vitro usefulness, to provide as much information about the differences and/or similarities between baby and adult skin permeability. The penetration characteristics of water through full-term baby, premature baby, and adult skin have been described by Fisher [13]. He described the in vitro barrier to water penetration of full-term baby to be the greatest, followed by adult, and that premature baby had almost no barrier at all. This paper expands his data to alcohols and fatty acids. All experimental designs contained one variable: the age of the skin.

MATERIALS AND METHODS

Skin Samples

All skin samples were obtained from autopsy. Abdominal samples were obtained from premature babies (26-28 weeks of gestation), full-term babies (38-40 weeks), and adults (18 years or older). Samples were frozen immediately and kept at $-70°C$ until just before use. A surface slice was taken from adult and full-term baby using a keratome (Storz Inst. Co., St. Louis, Missouri) set at 0.3 mm. Peeled whole epidermis, about 0.5 mm thick, was used from premature baby skin.

Penetration Cell and Collection System

The penetration cell is that reported by Fisher [13]. The major modification consists of automating the collection of 15 min samples by a fraction collector and a continuous flow system rather than a circulating reservoir. The flow rate of distilled water under the membrane was 2.0 ml/15 min. Samples were collected for 5-7 hr. The working diameter of the cell is 3 mm. The membrane (see below) is placed over the opening and held in place with a Teflon gasket and a threaded plug. The gasket and the plug have a 3 mm hole through their centers. The penetrant was deposited on the membrane through the above hole, after the water had been circulating for at least 15 min. At least 10 replicates were accumulated.

The effect of temperature on percutaneous penetration is known. Experiments were performed at room temperature with the assumption that relative penetration would be valid at higher body temperatures. However, when preliminary experiments indicated no detectable penetration of stearic acid in the full-term baby, with slight penetration in adult, and some penetration in premature, we decided that a more meaningful comparison could be made at $32°C$. Therefore the fatty acid series was all run in an incubator.

Table 1 Materials Employed in the Comparison of Skin Permeability

Penetrant	Specific activity (mCi/mmol)	Solvent	Amount applied (μl)	
Ethyl alcohol	4	–	0.9	μCi/30
Benzyl alcohol	8.65	–	5.5	μCi/5
Cetyl alcohol	4.48	Acetone	5.5	μCi/5
Decyl alcohol	15.2	–	6.25	μCi/5
Caprylic acid	2.62	Acetone	8	μCi/5
Lauric acid	12.5	Acetone	8	μCi/5
Oleic acid	55.96	Acetone	8	μCi/5
Stearic acid	50	Hexane	8	μCi/5

Model Membranes

Three additional materials were used: rat neonatal stratum corneum prepared by the method of Vinson [15], silastic medical grade polymer, and aluminum foil.

Application of the Test Molecules to the Membrane Surface

The materials listed in Table 1 were applied to the membrane surface with a microsyringe. Samples with more than 5 μL of solvent were gently dried with a stream of warm air. The syringe was positioned above, but not touching, the stratum corneum. The minimum 5-μL volume applied to the 0.07 cm^2 of membrane completely covered the surface and touched the Teflon gasket holding the skin in place.

Analysis of Data

The collection system delivered the effluent directly into scintillation vials. Each hour during a run, 15 ml of Packard Insta-gel liquid scintillation cocktail was added to the vials; they were counted using an Intertechnique SL-4000. After each experiment the Teflon gasket was placed in 17 ml of scintillation cocktail and counted. The amount of penetrant on the gasket was not considered part of the dose available for penetration. A volume of penetrant equal to that applied to the skin was counted to determine the dose for each set of cells. Quench correction was obtained using external standardization processed by an Intertechnique 5000 Microprocessor.

If a skin sample showed unusually high penetration in the first 2 hr of a run, the tissue was examined under a microscope for holes or imperfections at the end of the experiment. If an obvious defect existed, the data was not included. At the end of each experiment, the skin samples were incubated in 1 ml Packard Soluene at 37°C for 24 hr. Scintillation cocktail (16 ml) was added and the sample was counted.

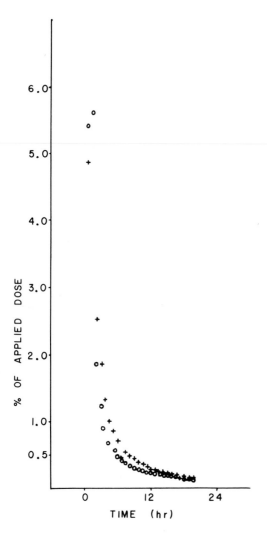

Figure 1   Penetration of 4.1 × 10⁶ cpm [¹⁴C] benzoic acid through silastic.

In all experiments, except the ethanol series, total recovery of the applied radioactively labeled material exceeded 95%.

RESULTS

Medical Grade Polymer (Dow)

Silastic medical grade polymer (#HH 1420) is used because of its permeability and consistency (Fig. 1) as an example of a solid material applied to an artificial membrane. Note the importance of the first few hours of the experiment. This is a case where the rate-limiting step is not penetration through the membrane, but transfer from the bulk of the material to the surface of the membrane. Materials were selected that did not exhibit this quality. Note the amount of variability in the system itself. The greatest variation seen using this nonbiological substrate is less than 1% in 10 cells. We therefore assume that variation seen in human data to be variation inherent from subject to subject and sample to sample.

Rat Neonatal Stratum Corneum

Figure 2 is a graphic representation of a second model membrane material, rat neonatal stratum corneum. With liquids, as long as the viscosity is not too great, there is usually no migration problem from the bulk to the membrane. In this case, an equilibrium is reached in the first hour; a pseudosteady state is maintained as long as the membrane surface is covered by a continuous film of penetrant.

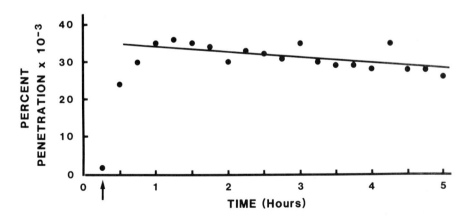

Figure 2   Penetration of $[^3H]H_2O$ through rat neonatal stratum corneum. Arrow (↑) indicates when the solution was applied.

Aluminum Foil

Penetration of volatile materials present an interesting challenge to studies of this type. Sealing the cell or placing a plug in the application hole was considered. A film over the top of the cell would allow vaporization above the skin surface; a plug could increase the pressure on the remaining air space above the skin and possibly exert some effect upon the penetration. We decided to leave the system open and represent the percentage of penetration as the average amount of penetrant on the skin for the 6-hr period.

Aluminum foil was placed under 10 skin samples to measure the evaporation of each penetrant. Distilled water was run under the cells with the radioactive material in place for 6 hr. The amount of material recovered at the end of the 6 hr from the cell, gasket, skin, and foil was determined. Ethyl alcohol was the only material that did not return more than 95% of the starting dose. The average amount of ethyl alcohol present for the 6-hr period was 33% of the applied

Table 2 Comparative Penetration of Alcohols Through Three Age Groups of Human Skin

	Adult	Full-term	Premature
Ethanol			
%, 6 hr	1.3	1.6	4.8
± SD	0.3	0.3	1.5
N	14	18	17
Lag time (min)	19	24	29
Benzyl alcohol			
%, 6 hr	1.42	0.73	35.5
± SD	0.94	0.48	5.6
N	16	12	14
Lag time (min)	25	33	15
Decanol			
%, 6 hr	0.0247	0.0158	0.259
± SD	0.0036	0.0057	0.057
N	10	10	10
Lag time (min)	23	35	3
Cetyl alcohol			
%, 6 hr	0.0045	0.0023	0.0418
± SD	0.001	0.002	0.03
N	11	11	14
Lag time (min)	0	0	2

dose. Therefore, the percentage dose penetration for ethyl alcohol has been adjusted for evaporation.

The Penetration of an Alcohol Series Through
Skin of Three Age Groups

The results of the study of the penetration of a series of alcohols through skin of three age groups are in Table 2 and Figures 3 to 6. The lag times shown are based on linear regression analysis of the data points obtained. The lag time in minutes is the point where the line generated intercepts the time axis. Lag time is considered an estimation of resistance to diffusion until a pseudo-steady state

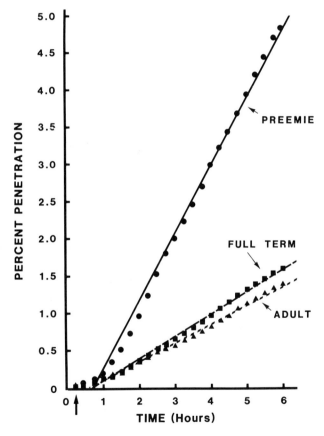

Figure 3 Cumulative penetration of [^{14}C] ethanol through three age groups of human skin. Arrow (↑) indicates when the solution was applied.

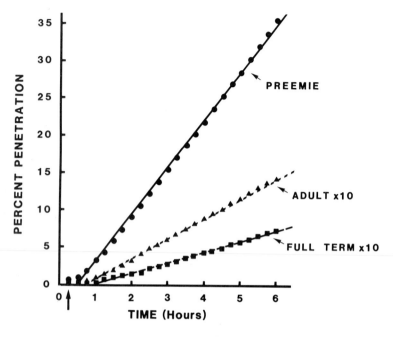

Figure 4 Cumulative penetration of [^{14}C] benzyl alcohol through three age groups of human skin. Arrow (↑) indicates when the solution was applied.

is achieved. Lag time is affected by many factors, but most importantly by barrier thickness, molecular size, and solubility.

With the nonvolatile alcohols, benzyl, cetyl, and decyl, penetration through skin of premature infants was consistently greater than through skin of adults. A maximum difference was discerned with benzyl alcohol where 1.4% of the applied dose penetrated through adult skin after 6 hr and 35.5% penetrated through premature skin after the same time. In general, twice as much material penetrated adult skin than full-term infant skin with the nonvolatile alcohols. However, total penetration after 6 hr never reached 2.0% of the applied dose with adult or full-term infant skin.

In contrast to the nonvolatile alcohols, ethanol showed comparable penetration after 6 hr through full-term infant and adult skin in vitro, 1.6 and 1.3%, respectively. Greater penetration was observed through premature skin (~3X) than through either adult or full-term infant; the differences were not as large as seen with the nonvolatile members of the series.

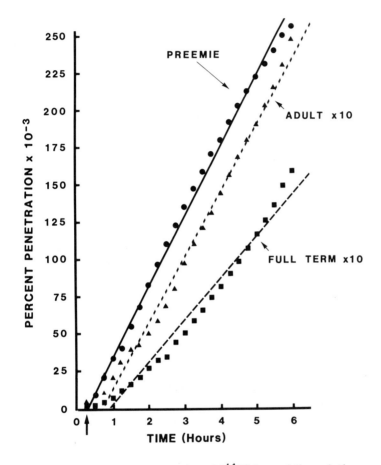

Figure 5 Cumulative penetration of [^{14}C] decanol through three age groups of human skin. Arrow (↑) indicates when the solution was applied.

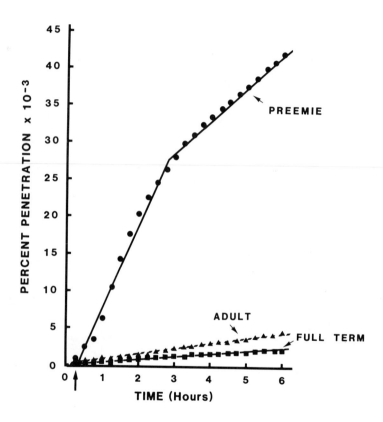

Figure 6 Cumulative penetration of [^{14}C] cetyl alcohol through three age groups of human skin. Arrow (↑) indicates when the solution was applied.

The Penetration of a Fatty Acid Series Through
Skin of Three Age Groups

Table 3 and Figures 7 to 10 summarize the penetration of a series of fatty acids. Penetration overall was slight compared to the alcohol series. With regard to the solid fatty acids, stearic acid showed little penetration through skin of the three age groups with no significant differences between them. Lauric acid showed a greater amount of penetration through skin than did stearic acid. The order of permeability of lauric acid through three age groups of skin was: premature, full-term, and adult with 0.648, 0.285, and 0.114% of the applied dose penetrating after 6 hr, respectively.

Caprylic acid showed the greatest amount of penetration of any liquid fatty

Table 3 Comparative Penetration of Fatty Acids Through Three Age Groups of Human Skin

	Adult	Full-Term	Premature	Dermis[a]
Caprylic Acid				
%, 6 hr	0.96	2.94	1.75	
± SD	0.81	0.60	0.99	
N	10	10	10	
Lag time (min)	40	40	42	
Oleic Acid				
%, 6 hr	0.0093	0.088	0.101	
± SD	0.0009	0.016	0.056	
N	10	10	10	
Lag time (min)	0	30	39	
Stearic Acid				
%, 6 hr	0.014	0.011	0.014	0.125
± SD	0.004	0.005	0.010	0.06
N	10	10	10	10
Lag time (min)	9	15	15	0
Lauric Acid				
%, 6 hr	0.114	0.285	0.648	
± SD	0.050	0.111	0.514	
N	10	10	10	
Lag time (min)	32	17	21	

[a]The value is an average of five adult and five full-term samples.

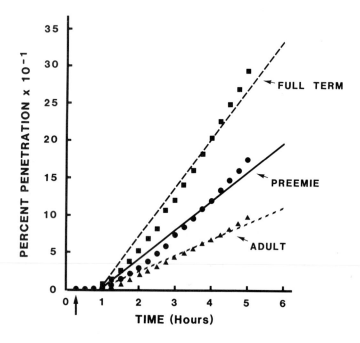

Figure 7 Cumulative penetration of [^{14}C] caprylic acid through three age groups of human skin. Arrow (↑) indicates when the solution was applied.

acid in the series. Values of 0.96, 2.94, and 1.75% of the applied dose after 6 hr were obtained for adult, full-term infant, and premature skin, respectively. Unlike the other fatty acids in the series, caprylic acid showed the greatest amount of penetration through full-term infant skin. In contrast, the more viscous oleic acid exhibited a penetration pattern similar to the nonvolatile alcohols: premature infant skin was more permeable than full-term infant skin which was less permeable than adult skin.

An experiment was conducted to discern the role of the dermis as a barrier to penetration to materials of low water solubility qualities, e.g., fatty acids. It has been hypothesized that the dermis may play a significant role in retarding penetration of such materials. The penetration of stearic acid through 0.5-mm adult and full-term infant dermis was determined (Table 3). Penetration of stearic acid through dermis of adult or full-term infant dermis was 10 times greater than through epidermis indicating the importance of the stratum corneum's role as a barrier to penetrants.

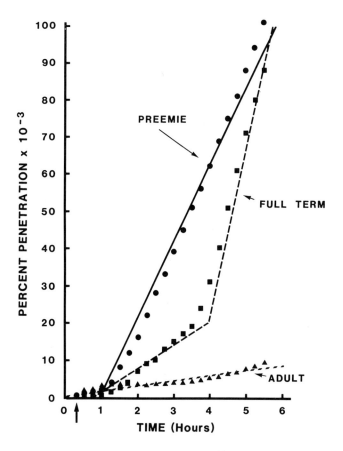

Figure 8 Cumulative penetration of [^{14}C] oleic acid through three age groups of human skin. Arrow (↑) indicates when the solution was applied.

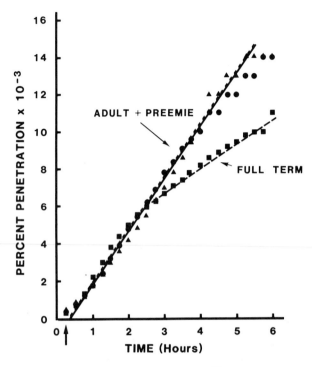

Figure 9 Cumulative penetration of [^{14}C] stearic acid through three age groups of human skin. Arrow (↑) indicates when the solution was applied.

DISCUSSION

This paper examined the question of the similarity of penetration through baby versus adult skin. Full-term baby skin, in this in vitro system, is generally an excellent barrier. The differences seen in penetration of some of the fatty acids is possibly due to their greater solubility in corneum lipids. As discussed by Sheuplien [11], solubility in corneum lipid would be a factor in skin penetration. Full-term baby skin samples stain heavier for lipid than adult samples (Fisher, personal communication). Therefore, it is not unreasonable that the liquid fatty acids penetrated the full-term baby skin slightly more than the adult skin. These data agree with those of Scheuplien and Blank who found that the lower molecular weight, less viscous, and more volatile substances are more apt to permeate the skin barrier [16].

There is often doubt that biological results are truly representative of percu-

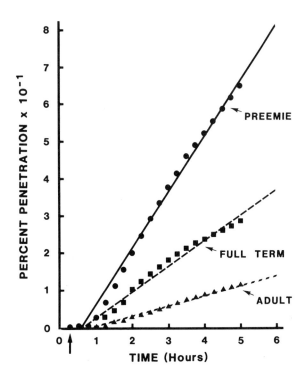

Figure 10 Cumulative penetration of [^{14}C]lauric acid through three age groups of human skin. Arrow (↑) indicates when the solution was applied.

taneous absorption, e.g., that measurement of blood or urine levels does not take into consideration metabolism or distribution elsewhere in the body. Attempts were made to reduce the testing variables that could interfere with the interpretation of the results. Prescreening the materials in a model system so that penetration through the barrier would be the rate-limiting step eliminated certain substances from consideration. Allowing for but not preventing evaporation allowed us to examine penetration of a type of molecule whose penetration characteristics should be of interest.

To fully understand the barrier of the newborn much additional investigation is required. Even if the penetration of a material is determined to be equal or less through full-term infant skin than in the adult caution must still be observed in application of that material to the infant. It must be noted that the ratio of surface area to body weight is greater in the infant than in older children and adults. Consequently, given similar amounts of penetration of a material through skin, the infant receives the largest dose on a weight-to-weight basis.

REFERENCES

1. Keipert JA: The absorption of topical corticosteroids with particular reference to percutaneous absorption in infancy and childhood. Med J Aust 1: 1021-1025, 1971.
2. Powell H, Swarner O, Gluck L, Lapert P: Hexachlorophene mylinopathy in premature infants. J Pediatr 82:976-981, 1973.
3. Feinblatt BI, Aceto T, Beckhorn G, Bruck E: Percutaneous absorption of hydrocortisone in children. Am J Dis Child 112:218-224, 1966.
4. Kagan BM, Mirman B, Calvin J, Lundeen E: Cyanosis in premature infants due to aniline dyes. J Pediatr 34:574-578, 1949.
5. Feiwel M: Percutaneous absorption of topical steroids in children. Br J Dermatol 81:[Suppl. 4] 113-116, 1969.
6. Shuman RM, Leech RW, Alvord EC: Neurotoxicity of hexachlorophene in humans, a clinicopathological study of 46 premature infants. Arch Neurol 32:320-325, 1975.
7. Armstrong RW, Eichner ER, Klein DE, Bartel WF, Bennett JV, Jonsson V, Bruce H, Loveless LE: Pentachlorophenol poisoning in a nursery for newborn infants. II. Epidemiologic and toxicologic studies. J Pediatr 75:317-325, 1969.
8. Brown BW: Fatal phenol poisoning from improperly laundered diapers. Am J Public Health 60:901-902, 1970.
9. Nachman RL, Esterley NB: Increased skin permeability in preterm infants. J Pediatr 79:628-632, 1971.
10. Wildnauer RH, Kennedy R: Transepidermal water loss of human newborns. J Invest Dermatol 54:483-486, 1970.
11. Scheuplein RJ: Mechanism of percutaneous adsorption I. Routes of penetration and the influence of solubility. J Invest Dermatol 45:334-346, 1965.
12. Franz TJ: Percutaneous absorption. On the relevance of in vitro data. J Invest Dermatol 64:190-195, 1975.
13. Fisher LB: The permeability of infant skin. Presented at the First Pediatric Dermatology Meeting, July 29, 1976.
14. Blank IH, Scheuplein RJ, MacFarlane DJ: Mechanism of percutaneous absorption. III. The effect of temperature on the transport of non-electrolytes across the skin. J Invest Dermatol 88:21-23, 1963.
15. Vinson LJ, Singer EJ, Koehler WR, Lehman MD, Masurat T: The nature of the epidermal barrier and some factors influencing skin permeability. Toxicol Appl Pharmacol 7:[Suppl. II] 7, 1965.
16. Scheulpein RJ, Blank IH: Permeability of the skin. Physiol Rev 51:702-709, 1971.
17. Scheuplein RJ, King PN: Solubility of organic molecules in the lipids of the stratum corneum. J Invest Dermatol 64:209, 1975.

MICROBIOLOGY

12

Bacteriology of Newborn Skin

JAMES J. LEYDEN
University of Pennsylvania, Philadelphia, Pennsylvania

Several workers have investigated the cutaneous bacterial flora of the neonatal period. Their focus has been mainly on the prevalence and factors involved in the development of infection. Skin infections, particularly of the umbilical cord stump and the circumcision site, were at one time a major medical problem and continue to occur in an episodic fashion.

There is agreement that at birth, relatively few organisms are found on human skin, but argument exists regarding the prevalence of these organisms on newborn skin. For example, Sarkany sampled the head, scapula, axilla, groin, and periumbilical areas with contact plates and found staphylococci in all babies, diphtheroids in 60%, coliform organisms in the diaper and umbilical areas, and occasional streptococci [1]. Four of five babies delivered by caesarean section were sterile with the fifth having scattered colonies of *Staphylococcus epidermidis*.

Evans et al. cultured the same five areas and the anterior nares by both contact plates and swabs approximately 2 hr after birth. *S. epidermidis* was recovered from 50 to 75% of skin sites and in 14% of the anterior nares and was by far the most commonly isolated organism. Gram-negative organisms, including *Escherichia coli* and *Proteus* species were found in less than 10% of infants and, when present, were usually in the groin and the axilla [2]. This study demonstrated a lack of correlation between recovery of organisms from infant skin and the microflora of the mothers vagina, suggesting that skin colonization results from contacts with nursery personnel and family members after delivery.

These workers also monitored the microflora of the umbilical cord and the

167

anterior nares for 6 consecutive days in nearly 1400 newborns [3]. *S. epidermidis* were recovered from the umbilical area in 28% of newborns on the first day of life, 40% on day 2, and then remained constant. Anterior nares cultures had *S. epidermidis* in 6% of infants on day 1, 26% on day 2, 45% on day 3, and then reached 50% for the remaining 3 days, suggesting that anterior nares colonization follows cutaneous colonization.

The most comprehensive study was that of McAllister et al. who cultured 1103 infants (the umbilical cord, nose, throat, groin, and rectum serving as sites) on days 1, 3, 5, 7, and then weekly for 5 weeks [4]. While their data are difficult to interpret because they are total numbers of bacterial isolates broken down into "pathogens" and "nonpathogens," cutaneous and anterior nares colonization increased significantly in the first 48 hr of life and tended to increase further for the first week and then level off.

Why the skin contains a paucity of organisms at birth is unknown. Sarkany and Gaylarde studied the effect of amniotic fluid on the growth of staphylococci and diptheroids and were unable to demonstrate any antibacterial properties [5]. Their work confirmed and extended an earlier report by Walsh et al. [6] and thus the scarcity of organisms on newborn skin appears not to be related to any antimicrobial action of amniotic fluid. The possibility that the vernix exerts an antimicrobal effect has not been studied. The absence of free fatty acids in that material makes this possibility less likely, however.

None of these studies employed quantitative techniques and their focus was mainly on the prevalence of colonization by pathogens particularly *S. aureus* and in elucidating the factors involved in determining colonization with *S. aureus* and subsequent infection. Repeated quantitative bacteriology facilitates the distinction of transient organisms from true residents because transients are normally found in relatively low numbers and are not found on repeated culturing. We sampled 25 newborns: all were healthy full-term infants, 12 boys and 13 girls, within 2 hr of birth and again on days one, 2, and 5 and finally at the first well-baby check, which was usually 6 weeks after birth. Quantitative cultures were obtained by the detergent scrub technique of Williamson and Kligman [7] from the axilla, groin, forehead, and antecubital fossa.

The results are summarized in Tables 1 and 2. At birth, aerobic bacteria are commonly found (76-80% of sites), but the total number of organisms was extremely low: 36-51 organisms/cm^2. Within 24 hr, organisms were recovered from all sites. The axillae and groin had 10^3 organisms/cm^2 compared to an average of 540 for the scalp. At 48 hr, the scalp had 525 organisms/cm^2, the axilla had an average of 10,120 organisms, and the groin contained 220,100. Virtually the same number of organisms were found in the groin and axilla at day 5, while the scalp had increased to an average of 2,730 organisms/cm^2. By

Table 1 Prevalence of Bacteria in 25 Newborns (%)

Day	CNC			S. aureus			GNB			P. acnes			Aerobic diphtheroids		
	Sc	Ax	Gr	Sc	Ax	Gr	Sc	Ax	Gr	Sc	Ax	Gr	Sc	Ax	Gr
0-1	80	76	76	0	0	0	0	4	16	28	4	8	8	0	0
2	100	100	100	0	4	12	4	12	16	40	0	4	8	4	8
5	100	100	100	4	4	4	0	24	40	20	0	0	12	12	16
42	100	100	100	0	0	0	4	12	40	28	16	16	12	12	16

CNC, coagulase-negative cocci; GNV, gram-negative bacteria; Sc, scalp; Ax, axilla; Gr, groin.

Table 2 Aerobic Flora in Newborns (total count/cm^2)[a]

	2-5 hr	24 hr	48 hr	5 days	6 weeks
Axilla (25)	42	4120	10,120	12,240	98,100
Scalp (25)	36	540	545	2,736	180,200
Groin (25)	51	2140	220,100	440,000	312,000

[a]Geometric mean count.

6 weeks, the total number of organisms for each site was comparable to that found in adults, with 180,200 organisms on the scalp, 98,100 in the axilla, and 312,000 on the groin. Coagulase-negative cocci were the most commonly found organism. Several strains were further studied and all proved to be *S. epidermis*. Surprisingly, diphtheroids were rarely recovered. The finding of only a very limited number of bacteria in the first hours of life indicates that newborn skin is essentially sterile at birth. The few organisms could easily result from either contact with nursery personnel, contact with their mothers, or even from contamination during the passage through the vagina. Within 48 hr, dense populations are found in the axilla and groin, possibly reflecting the onset of eccrine sweating and the effect of semiocclusion in intertriginous areas and, in the groin, the added occlusion provided by the diaper. By 6 weeks, the flora is quantitatively comparable to that of adults. The relative lack of diphtheroids was surprising and may reflect several factors, such as differences in substrate available in infant skin, our patient population, or the antiseptic practices of the nursery. Certainly the very low recovery of *S. aureus* reflects the latter which consisted of a daily gentle cleansing with 3% hexachlorophene.

NEONATAL CUTANEOUS INFECTION

Cutaneous infection in the neonate is due to *S. aureus* in the vast majority of cases. In the 1950s and early 1960s epidemics of neonatal superficial and deep tissue infection due to *S. aureus* were common. Many studies conducted during those years found a high incidence of *S. aureus* colonization of normal skin and in particular the umbilical cord stump. In 1953 Barber et al. reported 75% [8], Forfar found 60% [9], and Hurst found 99% of one series of 106 infants carried *S. aureus* [10]. In contrast to these strikingly high rates of recovery of *S. aureus* are the findings of Sarkany and Gaylarde of only occasional recovery of *S. aureus* [1], our failure to recover *S. aureus* in a small group of infants, and the recovery of small numbers of *S. aureus* from 2.6% of 963 umbilical cords and 4% of 838 anterior nares samples in the extensive study of McAllister et al. [4]. Presumably, these differences in recovery of *S. aureus* reflect the adoption of antiinfective measures such as the careful use of soaps containing hexachlorophene and strict adherence to policies of hand-washing between handling infants.

The factors involved in *S. aureus* colonization of infant skin and dissemination have been the subject of numerous rather elegant and complete studies. Gezon et al. showed that male infants have a higher rate of cutaneous infections than females and that this sex difference is not altered by antiinfective measures [11]. A probable contributing factor is circumcision which provides another wound (in addition to the umbilical cord stump) with its serous exudate and favorable environment for colonization by *S. aureus.* This possibility was further strengthened by their findings that males had pyodermas predominantly in the anterior diaper area while females showed no particular localization. In both sexes, the oozing, serous, umbilical stump was fertile for infection. They also demonstrated that skin colonization occurred prior to nasal colonization.

Nasal colonization is an important step in the spread of virulent strains of *S. aureus* from baby to baby and from baby to nursery personnel and then to other babies [12]. While nasal colonization was necessary for spread of *S. aureus,* equally important was contamination of the hands of nursery personnel. Spread of *S. aureus* appears to occur primarily via direct contact with contaminated hands rather than aerial dispersal. The recognition of these factors has resulted in antiinfective practices such as careful cleansing of the umbilical stump and circumcision site with antimicrobial substances such as hexachlorophene and more recently with chlorhexidine. These agents clearly are capable of significantly reducing the prevalences of *S. aureus* colonization and infection and, coupled with strict adherence of hand washing by nursery personnel, epidemics of *S. aureus* infection have been significantly curtailed.

Another approach which has been successfully employed in combating epidemics of *S. aureus* infections has been the use of the principle known as "bacterial interference." In this procedure, the anterior nares and the umbilicus of newborns were colonized with a "less virulent" strain of *S. aureus* (502A) which then competitively blocked colonization by more virulent strains such as 80/81 [13]. This procedure, however, has proven not to be entirely benign; in one series 17 of 50 infants developed a pyoderma due to the "less virulent" 502A strain [14]. An untried possible extension of this principle would be the deliberate implantation of resident *S. epidermidis* on the umbilical cord stump, skin, and anterior nares. The presence of *S. epidermidis* has been shown to interfere with the establishment of *S. aureus* infection in carefully monitored experimental infections in humans. *S. aureus* colonization of the anterior nares also appears to be impeded by the presence of *S. epidermidis* and diphtheroids.

DIAPER RASH

The neonate and the newborn in general are particularly prone to dermatitis in the diaper area. The belief that microorganisms play a central role in this extremely common condition is ancient. In the early 1900s, dermatologists came to view urinary ammonia as an important etiologic factor. When Cooke demonstrated in 1921 that an aerobic, gram-positive rod, *Brevibacterium ammoniagenes*, was capable of liberating ammonia from urea, this organism came to be viewed as the etiologic agent [15]. In fact, diaper dermatitis is commonly referred to as "ammoniacial dermatitis." More recent studies have centered on the role of *Candida albicans*. *C. albicans* is frequently recovered, prevalence rates of up to 75% having been reported [16].

We investigated the role of microorganisms from several points of view. Quantitative cultures, as described above, were obtained from 40 infants from the inguinal fold, the thigh (within the area covered by diapers), the perineum, and perianal area. These infants were free of any signs of diaper dermatitis and had no history of previous episodes of dermatitis. The results are summarized in Table 3. The microflora of the diaper area ranged from 10^4 to 10^5 organisms/ cm^2. Coagulase-negative cocci were present in nearly every site and represented from 50 to 73% of the total flora. We made only limited attempts to classify these organisms further: the majority were *S. epidermidis*. Aerobic diphtheroids, particularly lipophilic strains, were commonly found and when present constituted 25-36% of the total numbers of organisms. Large-colony diphtheroids were less common and were found in approximately 20-30% of sites. When present, they constituted a small percentage of the total flora with the exception of six cases where they represented 55% of the total flora. At the time of these studies, the appreciation that aerobic diphtheroids on human skin fall into both *Corynebacterium* and *Brevibacterium* genera had not occurred. We have reexamined several of these strains and would tentatively classify lipophilic diphtheroids as *Corynebacteria* on the basis of the presence of corynomyocolic acid on gas chromatography analysis and the failure to produce methanethiol on incubation with L-methionine. Large colony diphtheroids can be either *Corynebacteria* or *Brevibacteria*. We obtained a strain of *Brevibacterium ammoniagenes* from the American Type Culture Center and found it to display a large, wrinkled, yellow colony on Trypticase Soy Agar; it was nonfluorescent, strongly urease-positive, and its growth was not enhanced by lipids. We found no similar organisms on the diaper area skin of these 40 infants.

We then quantitatively cultured the organisms present in the urine of the first diaper change in the morning. This was done in 18 infants diagnosed as having "ammoniacal dermatitis" by pediatricians caring for in-patients at the Childrens' Hospital of Philadelphia. Similar cultures were obtained from 63 infants free of any signs of diaper dermatitis. One milliliter aliquot was diluted in 0.05% buffered Triton-X-100 and then drop-plated in multiple media. The organisms recurred were then subcultivated and transferred onto standard urea slants. The presence of ammonia was graded on a 0 to +3 scale at 4-6 hr and after 24 hr on

Table 3 Microflora of Diaper Area in Normal Infants

	Inguinal fold (N = 40)	Thigh (N = 32)	Perineum (N = 30)	Perianal area (N = 30)
Geometric mean aerobic count/cm^2	240,000	92,400	892,300	610,000
Coagulase negative cocci[a]	38 (70)	31 (65)	30 (73)	29 (50)
Lipophilic diphtheroids	20 (25)	16 (32)	10 (29)	11 (36)
Large-colony diphtheroids	10 (16)	6 (55)	12 (35)	3 (55)
Gram-negative bacilli	32 (2)	28 (2)	29 (1.5)	27 (23.5)
C. albicans	0	0	3 (0.01)	0

[a]Number of positive sites, percentage of total flora in parenthesis.

Source: Leyden JJ, Kligman AM. The role of microorganisms in diaper dermatitis. Arch Dermatol 114:56-59, 1978. Copyright 1978, American Medical Association.

Table 4 Urine Microorganisms and Ammonia Production

	Number of isolates		Ammonia production	
	Rash	No rash	4-6 hr	24 hr
Coagulase negative *micrococcaceae*	7/18	43/63	10	33
S. aureus	1/18	1/63	0	0
Aerobic diphtheroids	13/18	42/63	12	18
Lactose-dermenting gram-negative rods	6/18	22/63	8	19
E. coli	5/18	25/63	0	0
Proteus	4/18	10/63	11	14
Pseudomonas	6/18	4/63	0	0
C. albicans	9/18	0/63	0	0

Source: Leyden JJ, Katy S, Stewart R, Kligman AM. Urinary ammonia and ammonia-producing microorganisms in infants with and without diaper dermatitis. Arch Dermatol 113:1678-1680, 1977. Copyright 1977, American Medical Association.

the basis of the intensity and extent of color changes. At the same time we measured the amount of ammonia present in the urine of the first diaper change in 26 infants with "ammoniacal dermatitis" (the above 18 infants were included) and in 82 infants free of diaper rash. One milliliter of each sample was diluted to 100 ml distilled water and free ammonia was measured by a pH meter with an ammonia-sensing electrode after addition of 10 M sodium hydroxide.

In 26 infants with diaper rash, the mean free ammonia concentration in the morning diaper was 40% ppm compared to 465 ppm in those free of any rash (a nonsignificant difference). Exposure of urine to jack bean urease to produce the maximal concentration of ammonia resulted in a mean of 7803 ppm in the diaper rash group and 7566 ppm in those free of rash.

Table 4 summarizes the prevalence of various organisms in the diapers of 18 infants with dermatitis and in 63 normals. There were no significant differences between the groups except for the recovery of *C. albicans* in nine of 18 with rash. The organisms capable of liberating ammonia included the *Micrococcacceae*. arobic diphtheroids, lactose fermenting gram-negative rods, and *Proteus* and *Pseudomonas*. The finding of a strong ammonia-producing organism did not correlate with the presence of diaper dermatitis. Rapid production of ammonia (4-6 hr) was present in eight of 18 infants with rash and in 33 of 63 without a

Table 5 Ammonia Production by Bacteria in Diaper Area

	4-6 hr			24 hr		
	+[a]	++	+++	+	++	+++
No rash (63)	14	16	3	20	32	17
Diaper dermatitis (18)	4	4	0	6	4	2

[a]Measurement made on standard urea slants containing phenol red indicator. + indicates less than 25% of tube showed color change; ++ indicates 25% to 50% of tube showed color change; +++ indicates 75% or more of the tube showed color change.

rash. After 24 hr, two infants with rash showed a +3 production of ammonia, four had a +2, and six a +1 production compared to 17 of 63 normals with a +3, 32 with a +2, and 20 with a +1 reaction (Table 5).

These studies argue against the concept that ammonia-producing organisms play an important etiologic role in the production of diaper dermatitis. No significant differences in either the prevalence of organisms capable of liberating ammonia or the rapidity with which ammonia was generated were found in those with and without diaper rash. Nor were any significant differences in ammonia concentration found in the two study groups. In further experiments, occlusive patch tests with ammoniacal solutions well in excess of that found in infant diapers, (the test concentration was 16,320 ppm) failed to induce erythema after a 24-hr exposure to infant buttock skin and also failed to induce damage after repeated application to the volar forearm of volunteers. All these results lead us to conclude that ammonia is not an important etiological factor in the *induction* of diaper rash. We also investigated whether the concentration of ammonia found in infant diapers might damage skin in a subclinical fashion and make it more susceptible to frictional injury. The friction required to induce visible erythema and superficial erosion was evaluated on the volar forearms of five volunteers on normal dry skin, skin exposed for 24 hr to a gauze pad saturated with filtered urine containing either 500 ppm ammonia or 20,000 ppm, and a site exposed for 24 hr to a water-saturated gauze pad. Erythema and erosions were produced significantly more easily in the skin exposed to water or either concentration of ammonia than in dry skin, but no significant difference was seen in sites exposed to water and those exposed to ammoniacal solutions.

We concluded that ammonia-producing organisms were not a significant etiological factor in the induction of diaper rash. The concentration of ammonia produced in infant skin is sufficient to be readily recognized by the human nose but insufficient to produce disease.

In the final experiment, we quantitatively cultured the diaper rash in 100 infants in an attempt to correlate clinical varieties with bacteriological results. These infants were classified clinically into the following categories: chafing dermatitis (20%), atopic dermatitis (24%), moniliasis (25%), moniliasis with disseminated "id" (15%), seborrheic dermatitis (10%), psoriasis (2%), and undecided (4%). The criteria for these diagnoses were as follows: (1) Chafing dermatitis: the eruption was present only in the diaper area, mainly where friction was greatest: the inner surfaces of the thighs, genitals, buttocks, and the abdomen. This form tends to wax and wane quickly, consisting of a mild erythema with a shiny glazed surface and occasional papules. (2) Atopic dermatitis: a variable inflammatory rash not diagnostic in itself, but with typical lesions of atopic dermatitis on the cheeks, neck, antecubital fossa, or extremities, along with a family history of atopic dermatitis, allergic rhinitis, or asthma. (3) Moniliasis: the diaper area showed a confluent intense erythema with a sharp border beyond which were satellite papules and pustules. Patients with this form of diaper dermatitis who subsequently developed a disseminated eruption consisting of discrete plaques of erythema and scaling on the trunk, extremities, neck, and scalp were classified as moniliasis with "id" reaction. (4) Seborrheic dermatitis: the diaper area showed erythema and scaling, most pronounced in the groin and buttocks creases, along with similar lesions in the retroauricular neck, axillary, and limb creases, as well as the scalp. (5) Psoriasis: well-marginated plaques of erythema with a heavy scale in the diaper area as well as the trunk and scalp, in addition to a family history of psoriasis.

No patient had received any therapy for at least 1 week prior to this study.

Cultures were obtained from as many as the following areas as possible: the inguinal fold, the anterior thigh (within the area covered by the diaper), the labia major, the perianal areas, and the buttocks. Samples for quantitative microbiological analysis were obtained by the detergent scrub technique of Williamson and Kligman [7]. In brief, this technique employs two 1-min scrubbings with 0.1% octoxynol-9 (Triton X-100) in a 3.8 cm^2 area of skin outlined by a sterile glass cylinder. Samples are pooled, serially diluted in half-strength, buffered Octoxynol-9, and then drop-plated onto trypticase soy agar (TSA) with lecithin and polysorbate 80, MacConkey's selective agar for gram-negatives, and Sabouraud's agar. Organisms were identified by standard techniques. The *Micrococcaceae* were identified only to the point of separating coagulase-positive *S. aureus*. Diphtheroids were sorted out into two groups: lipophilic diphtheroids whose growth is stimulated by lipids, and large-colony diphtheroids with large colonies that are not enhanced by lipids. Cooke's strain, *B. ammoniagenes* (an aerobic, short, gram-positive, nonmotile, non-spore-forming organism), was obtained from the American Type Culture Center (ATCC). On TSA it displays a large wrinkled, yellow colony; it is nonfluorescent, strongly urease-positive, and its growth is not enhanced by lipids. These characteristics would classify it as a large-colony diphtheroid. We considered an organism to be *B. ammoniagenes* is it had similar morphology to the ATCC strain and the urea-splitting test was strongly positive. *Candida albicans* was identified on the basis of germ tube formation in serum incubated at 37°C for 2 hr.

In those with diaper dermatitis, the geometric mean aerobic density was in the range of 10^5 organisms/cm^2 for all cases for all sites (Table 6). Thus, the density was approximately the same as in normals for the perineum, perianal, and inguinal fold areas but was higher for the thigh and labia. As in the latter, coagulase-negative cocci were present in nearly every case; similarly, lipophilic and large-colony diphtheroids were also frequently present in high numbers. Gram-negatives were very common, usually in small amounts. *Candida albicans* was present in 80% of those cases considered to be local moniliasis and in a third of those diagnosed as moniliasis with disseminated id. In seborrheic dermatitis, *C. albicans* was recovered in 20%. In all these instances it made up only 1-4% of the microflora. *Staphylococcus aureus* was also frequently isolated, in approximately 50% of the cases. Unlike *C. albicans*, it comprised a significant portion of the population, from 10 to 80%. Atopic dermatitis had the highest prevalence of *S. aureua* (100%), and its abundance was great, comprising on the average 80% of the microflora. Frequently it was the sole organism. Among the large-colony diphtheroids, *B. ammoniagenes* was recovered only six times.

Diaper dermatitis is not a specific diagnosis and is best viewed as a family of disorders. It is a regional diagnosis, such as "hand dermatitis," that has many different causes. Previous surveys have usually not correlated clinical findings with microbiology. Some discounted bacterial findings altogether, others see *C. albicans* as the culprit, while perhaps the view with greatest currency is that ammonia liberated from urea irritates the skin.

The most prevalent form of diaper dermatitis is the least serious, the shiny erythema on friction surfaces that produces an irritated or chafed look. This form comes and goes, affects most infants at some time, and responds quickly to simple drying measures and frequent diaper changes. Chafing rash is mild, and mothers generally do not seek medical help although pediatricians see this type not infrequently. Chafing dermatitis is usually not included in microbiological surveys, Brookes et al.'s [17] study being an exception since their sample was derived from a well-baby clinic. Like them, we could find no qualitative differences in those with and without chafing dermatitis, except for low numbers of *S. aureus*, which were found in 50% of such cases. The level of *S. aureus* was far below the 10^6/cm^2 we have established as the level at which an underlying dermatitis is truly secondarily infected.

Table 6 Prevalence of Microorganisms in Relation to Clinical Diagnosis

Clinical diagnosis	N	Aerobic density/cm²[a]	% of Positive samples (% of total flora when present)						
			C. albicans	S. aureus	GNR	LCD	LD	CNM	B. ammoniagenes
Moniliasis (satellite pustules)	25	764,500	80(4)	30(25)	60(11)	20(10)	40(20)	100(30)	0(0)
Moniliasis (disseminated "id")	15	932,000	33(2)	60(40)	50(20)	18(15)	22(10)	100(13)	0(0)
Atopic dermatitis	24	980,000	0(0)	100(80)	20(1)	5(2)	20(1)	100(16)	3(1)
Seborrheic dermatitis	10	732,000	20(1.5)	80(30)	40(3)	20(30)	10(10)	100(25)	0(0)
Psoriasis	2	487,000	0(0)	50(10)	100(1)	50(6)	50(11)	100(70)	1(2)
Chafing dermatitis	20	643,000	0(0)	50(20)	25(10)	20(3)	40(6)	100(60)	2(1)

[a]Geometric mean count.

GNR, gram-negative rods; LCD, large-colony diphtheroids; LD, lipophilic diphtheroids; CNM, coagulase-negative micrococcaceae.

Source: Leyden JJ, Kligman AM: The role of microorganisms in diaper dermatitis. Arch Dermatol 114:56-59, 1978. Copyright 1978, American Medical Association.

In those cases diagnosed as atopic dermatitis on the basis of typical lesions elswhere and the presence of a family history of atopic disease, *S. aureus* was found in all 24 and was the predominant organism, constituting 80% of the flora. These results are identical with our earlier findings in atopic dermatitis of other body areas of children [18]. We consider that *S. aureus* is a secondary invader in atopic dermatitis and contributes to morbidity when the density exceeds 10^6 organisms/cm^2 [18,19]. This figure probably is accurate for atopic dermatitis in the diaper area.

Likewise, the microflora in psoriatic diaper rash correspond to our findings in psoriasis of adults [20]. *Staphylococcus aureus* occurred in 50% of the cases but in low numbers (10% of the total flora). At this low density *S. aureus* is unlikely to play a significant role.

The findings in seborrheic dermatitis were mixed. In two of 10 cases, *C. albicans* was isolated. Both of these cases and six others also contained *S. aureus* at moderately high levels (30% of the total aerobic flora). *Candida albicans* has been recovered in other series of seborrheic dermatitis and has been viewed as a secondary aggravating factor [21]. Our cases are too few to lead to a firm conclusion. Our experimental experiences with *C. albicans* lead us to believe that its virulence is high and that is often an instigating factor rather than a secondary invader [22,23].

In cases diagnosed as moniliasis, recovery of the organism depends strongly on the clinical type. The recovery rate was 80% in typical local moniliasis. In more severe varieties with disseminated lesions, the recovery was much lower (33%). In both types *Candida* represented only a minor proportion of the total flora (2-4%). We recovered *C. albicans* in only five of 145 cultures from normal infant skin. When present, it represented less than 0.01% of the total flora. Dixon et al. [21] also found *C. albicans* to be extremely infrequent on normal skin (one of 68 cases); Brookes et al. found no *C. albicans* in 35 normal infants [17]. In contrast to these reports is the recovery rate of 12% from normal skin by Montes et al. [16]. Quantitative data for *C. albicans* were not given by Montes et al. or Brookes et al.; hence, it is known whether the density was as low as in our five cases. Failure to find *Candida* in clinically typical moniliasis and its recovery from other cases not suspected to be moniliasis helps sustain the prevailing view that *C. albicans* acts as a secondary aggravating factor but does not instigate the rash. Dixon et al. [21] found *C. albicans* in 63% of suspected cases and in 25% of those labeled "*Candida* unlikely." The recovery of *C. albicans* from severe diaper dermatitis with a dessiminated id has been quite variable. Jefferson [24] found *C. albicans* in 20 of 32 patients, and Ferguson et al. [25] reported almost a 50% incidence in 29 patients. On the other hand, Warin and Faulknes [26] found *Candida* in only four of 17 similar cases. Again, our quantitative data in this study do not settle this question either. When present, *C. albicans* made up only a small fraction of the flora. One should not be tempted to dismiss *C. albicans* on this account. Previous studies from our laboratory have shown that, in experimental induction of *Candida* infections, *C. albicans* represents only a minor percentage of the total flora (usually around 1%) [22,23]; in contrast to *S. aureus* in atopic dermatitis, where levels of $10^6/cm^2$ are required to aggravate preexisting dermatitis [18], $10^4/cm^2$ levels of *C. albicans* will promptly induce a primary dermatitis. Furthermore, in experimentally induced erosio interdigitalis blastomycetia, after initial breakdown of the skin, *C. albicans* becomes less and less frequently recovered and may disappear altogether even though the clinical reaction is progressive. The lower recovery rate from the most severe clinical cases and the low percentage of the total flora when present are in accord with the data from serial analysis of experimental *C. albicans* infections. These observations have led us to conclude that *C. albicans* plays a primary instigating role in certain severe forms of diaper rash. When recovered, it represents a significant finding and treatment directed against *Candida* is indicated.

REFERENCES

1. Sarkany I, Gaylarde CC: Skin flora of the newborn. Lancet i:589, 1967.
2. Evans HE, Akpata SO, Baki A: Relationship of the birth canal to the bacterial flora of the neonatal respiratory tract and skin. Obstet Gynecol 37: 94, 1971.
3. Evans HE, Akpata SO, Baki A: Factors influencing the establishment of the neonatal bacterial flora. Arch Environ Health 21:514, 1970.
4. McAllister TA, Givan J, Turner MJ, Kerr MM, Hutchinson, JH: The natural history of bacterial colonization of the newborn in a maternity hospital. Scot Med J 19:119, 1974.
5. Sarkany I, Gaylarde CC: The effect of amniotic fluid in bacterial growth. Br J Dermatol 80:241, 1968.
6. Walsh H, Hildbrant RJ, Prystowsky H: Growth inhibition factors in amniotic fluid. Am J Obstet Gynecol 93:590, 1965.
7. Williamson P, Kligman AM: A new method for the quantitative investigation of cutaneous bacteria. J Invest Dermatol 45:498, 1965.
8. Barber M, Wilson BD, Ripper JE, Williams REO: Spread of staphylococcus aureus in maternity department in absence of severe sepsis.
9. Forfar JO, Balf CL, Elias-James Edmunds TF: Staphylococcal infection of newborns. Br Med J 2:170, 1953.
10. Hurst V: Staphylococcal aureus in the infant upper respiratory tract. 1. Observations on hospital born babies. 2. Observations on dormicilary delivered babies. J Hygiene 55:229; 313, 1957.
11. Gezon HM, Thompson DJ, Yee RB, Rogers KD: Host factors in infection and disease in the newborn, in *Skin Bacteria and Their Role in Infection*, edited by Maibach HI, Hildick-Smith G. McGraw-Hill, New York, 1965.

12. Hurst V: Transmission of hospital staphylococci among newborn infants. Pediatrics 25:204, 1960.
13. Shinefield HR, Ribble JC, Boris M, Eichenwald HF: Bacterial interference; its effect on nursery-acquired infection with *Staphylococcus aureus*. Am J Dis Child 105:646, 1963.
14. Blair EB, Tull AH: Multiple infections among newborns resulting from colonization with *Staphylococcus aureus* 502A. Am J Clin Pathol 52:42, 1968.
15. Cooke JV: Dermatitis of the diaper region in infants (Jacquet dermatitis). Arch Dermatol Syphilol 14:539-546, 1921.
16. Montes LF, Pittillo RF, Hunt D, Narkates AJ, Dillon HC: Microbial flora in infants' skin: Comparison of types of micro-organisms between normal skin and diaper dermatitis. Arch Dermatol 103:640-645, 1971.
17. Brookes DB, Hubbert RM, Sarkany I: Skin flora of infants with napkin rash. Br J Dermatol 85:250-254, 1971.
18. Leyden JJ, Marples RR, Kligman AM: Staphylococcus aureus in lesions of atopic dermatitis. Br J Dermatol 90:525-530, 1974.
19. Leyden JJ: Antibiotic usage in dermatological practice. Int J Dermatol 13:342-352, 1974.
20. Marples RR, Heaton CL, Kligman AM: Staphylococcus aureus in psoriasis. Arch Dermatol 107:568-570, 1973.
21. Dixon PN, Warin RP, English MP: Rose of candida albicans infection in napkin rashes. Br Med J 2:23-27, 1969.
22. Rebora A, Marples RR, Kligman AM: Experimental Candida albicans infection. Arch Dermatol 108:69-73, 1973.
23. Rebora A, Marples RR, Kligman AM: Erosio interdigitalis blastomycetica. Arch Dermatol 108:66-68, 1973.
24. Jefferson J: Napkin psoriasis. Br J Dermatol 78:614-615, 1966.
25. Fergusson AG, Fraser NG, Grant PW: Napkin dermatitis with psoriasiform ide: A review of 52 cases. Br J Dermatol 78:289-296, 1966.
26. Warin RP, Faulkner KE: Napkin psoriasis. Br J Dermatol 73:445-447, 1961.

13

Adherence of *Staphylococcus aureus* to Infant and Adult Nasal Mucosal Cells

RAZA ALY, HENRY R. SHINEFIELD, and HOWARD MAIBACH
University of California Medical School, San Francisco, California

The skin of the newborn at birth is physiologically different from that of the adult, including a coating with vernix caseosa and an elevated pH of about 7.4 [1]. The more neutral pH may be more conducive to microbial multiplication than the somewhat acid skin pH of adults [2]. The human fetus is normally bacteriologically sterile as evidenced by negative cultures obtained at the time of elective cesarean section. By the end of the first fortnight, the infant has acquired most of the organisms found on the corresponding areas of the adult. Differences are mainly quantitative, but a few qualitative differences are noted.

Gillespie et al. [3] were the first to study the sequence in which various anatomical sites of the infant become colonized. The umbilical cord was usually colonized with *Staphylococcus aureus* before the nose; the groin acquired staphylococci almost at the same time as the cord.

Bacterial colonization in the oral cavity of the human is low during the first day after birth, increasing to the adult level on day 3 [4,5]. The reason for this paucity of bacteria during early neonatal life has not been fully explained. Ofek et al. [5] reported that the adherence capacity of groups A and B streptococci to buccal mucosal cells at birth (day 1) was minimal and rapidly increased toward the adult level on day 3.

Adherence of microorganisms to the skin surface is one factor which determines their colonization. Not all bacteria adhere to skin even when competition from other bacteria is eliminated [6]. The capacity of a given microorganism to colonize a particular epithelial surface is proportional to the ability of the organism to adhere to that surface. Group A streptococci isolated from skin adhere in greater numbers to human skin epithelial cells than to cells obtained from buccal mucosa, whereas streptococci isolated from the throat tend to adhere better to buccal epithelial cells [7]. *S. aureus* vary in their ability to attach to nasal epithelial cells [3]. Nasal *S. aureus* carriers have a greater affinity for *S. aureus* than do noncarriers.

We investigated the adherence of *S. aureus* to nasal mucosal cells in newborns and compared this to the binding capacity of the adult epithelial cells. We chose nasal epithelial cells because the nose is an important reservoir for *S. aureus.*

MATERIALS AND METHODS

Healthy infants were selected. Nasal epithelial cells were obtained on days 1-5 after birth. Corresponding samples were collected from adults for comparisons.

Collection of Samples

Nasal epithelial cells were collected from infants and adults by gently scraping epithelia from the anterior nares with a wooden sterile applicator by methods previously described [6].

Preparation of Bacteria and Nasal Mucosal Cells

S. aureus was grown in trypticase soy broth, washed three times in phosphate buffer, and resuspended at about 10^8 organisms/ml for the adherence experiment. Mucosal cell preparation and bacterial suspensions (1 ml each) were mixed and incubated at 35°C for 90 min. After incubation the cells were washed free of unattached bacteria on an 8-μm filter, using 40 mil 0.075 M sodium phosphate buffer. Direct smears were prepared from each epithelial cell suspension and stained for 15 sec with Gram's crystal violet. The bacteria adhering to epithelial cells were examined under the light microscope. Control epithelial cell suspensions were incubated with phosphate buffer (without bacteria) to determine the number of bacteria already adhering to the cells.

RESULTS

Adult nasal epithelial cells treated with *S. aureus* are shown in Figure 1A. The average number of *S. aureus* adhering to adult epithelial cells was 67 ± 70. Mucosal cells incubated with phosphate buffer but not with bacteria served as the control (Fig. 1B).

Attachment of *S. aureus* to nasal mucosal cells of infants and adults was compared (Table 1). The binding of *S. aureus* by nasal epithelial cells was markedly

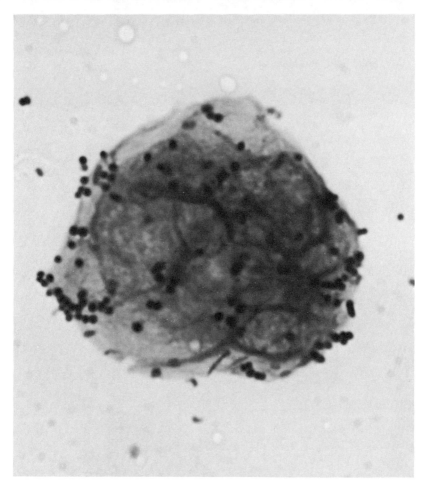

Figure 1A Adult nasal epithelial cell mixed with *S. aureus*.

Table 1 Adherence of *S. aureus* to Nasal Epithelial Cells from Newborns of Various Ages

Age (days)	% of adherence[a]	P
1	22	<0.001
2	25	0.001
3	38	0.001
4	35	0.001
5	98	>0.873

[a]Adherence of *S. aureus* to adult nasal mucosal cells was considered 100%.
Fifty epithelial cells were counted for each age group.

Source: Ref. 8. Copyright 1980, American Medical Association.

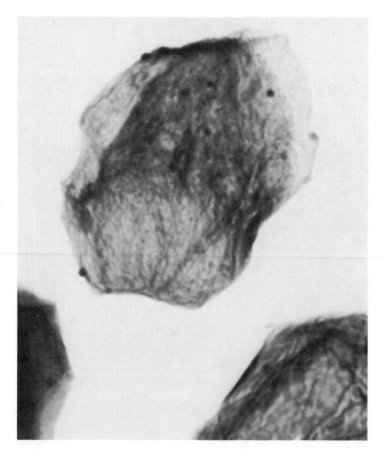

Figure 1B Adult nasal epithelial cell not mixed with *S. aureus* (control).

less on day 1 (P < 0.001) remaining at a low level until day 4 (P < 0.001). On day 5, the *S. aureus* binding to epithelial cells reached the adult level. There was no significant difference in adherence between the adult and the day 5 infant nasal mucosal cells (P > 0.873).

DISCUSSION

For certain bacteria, particularly *S. aureus,* the nose is the primary site of multi plication and dissemination. By reducing nasal staphylococci, a rapid reduction of skin and environmental staphylococci occurs [9]. With the present in vitro model utilizing isolated nasal mucosal cells and bacteria, the host-parasite relationship can be closely studied.

We have demonstrated that the ability of nasal epithelial cells to bind to *S. aureus* is markedly low during the first 4 days of life reaching adult levels on the 5th day. Ofek et al. [5] showed that the binding of buccal epithelial cells to streptococci group A and B was minimal on day 1 and 2 and reached the maximal level on day 3. The failure of bacteria to adhere to the mucous membrane of newborns may be due to the immature receptor sites or other host local factors. Streptococci binding appears to be due to lipoteichoic acid located on the surface of the organisms [4,5]. Teichoic acid, a component of *S. aureus* cell wall, mediates the binding of these organisms to nasal mucosal cells [10]. Knowledge about the receptor sites of infant epithelial cells for staphylococcal binding is lacking. Nasal colonization of the infant with *S. aureus* usually follows staphylococcal colonization of other body sites [11].

A better understanding of the mechanisms involved in the attachment of *S. aureus* to infant nasal epithelial cells should provide useful information regarding colonization of newborn mucous membranes and help clarify how this differs from that of the older infant and adult. It remains to be determined whether this information will lead to more effective methods of eradicating *S. aureus* colonization in either group.

REFERENCES

1. Behrendt H, Green M: Skin pH pattern in the newborn infant. Am J Dis Child 95:35-41, 1958.
2. Aly R, Shirley C, Cunico B, Maibach HI: Effect of prolonged occlusion on the microbial flora, pH, CO_2 and transepidermal water loss on human skin. J Invest Dermatol 71:378-381, 1978.
3. Gillespie WA, Simpson K, Tozer RC: Staphylococcal infection in a maternity hospital. Lancet 2:1075-1080, 1958.
4. Beachey EH: Binding of group A streptococci to human oral mucosal cells by lipoteichoic acid. Trans Assoc Am Physician 88:285-292, 1975.
5. Ofek I, Beachey EH, Jefferson W, Campbell GL: Cell membrane binding properties of group A streptococcal lipoteichoic acid. J Exp Med 141:990-1003, 1975.
6. Aly R, Shinefield HR, Strauss WG, Maibach HI: Bacterial adherence to nasal mucosal cells. Infect Immun 17:546-549, 1977.
7. Alkan M, Ofek I, Beachey EH: Adherence of pharyngeal and skin strains of group A streptococci to human skin and oral epithelial cells. Infect Immun 18:555-557, 1977.
8. Aly R, Shinefield HR, Maibach HI: Adherence of Staphylococcus aureus to infant nasal epithelial cells. Am J Dis Child 134:522-523, 1980.
9. White A, Smith J: Nasal reservoir as the source of extranasal staphylococci. Antimicrob Agents Chemother 1963:679-683, 1964.

10. Aly R, Shinefield HR, Litz C, and Maibach HI: Role of teichoic acid in the binding of *Staphylococcus aureus* to nasal epithelial cells. J Infect Dis 141:463-465, 1980.
11. Hurst V: Colonization of bacteria in the newborn, in *Skin Bacteria and Their Role in Infection,* edited by Maibach HI, Hildick-Smith G. McGraw-Hill, New York, 1964, pp 127-141.

TOXICOLOGY

14

Diaper Dermatitis and the Role of Predisposition

EDWARD K. BOISITS and JOHN J. McCORMACK

Johnson and Johnson Baby Products Company, Skillman, New Jersey

The term "eczema" is perplexing to those not familiar with the capriciousness of the word's usage. It may even have different meanings in American and European literature. Some consider the term to be synonymous with "dermatitis." Many consider it useful to think of eczema as a "genus" of skin disorder, and less specific than one of its "species," for example, atopic eczema [1]. Dermatitis, without a qualifying adjective, is a less definite term since it simply refers to an inflammation of the skin which may result in a spectrum of lesions varying from acute necrosis and ulceration to simple erythema. A comparison of some "species" of "eczema" is shown in Table 1.

Lesions of eczema may have a transitory or spatial relationship to each other: a lesion may evolve from one stage to another or several stages may be present simultaneously on different parts of the body.

There are four phases of eczema, any one of which may persist as the dominant feature depending on the age of the patient, the local physiologic characteristics of the skin involved, and the persistence of the underlying cause. The initial stage (1) is erythema which proceeds to (2) formation of microvesicles and weeping or oozing. The epidermal response to the injurious process then causes a burst of rapid epidermal mitotic activity which leads to (3) scaling. Finally, (4) lichenification (thickening of the skin with increased visibility of normal skin makrings) and pigmentary disturbances (usually, an initial increase followed by decrease in pigmentation) supervene. In the young infant, the first three stages predominate and lichenification is not seen.

Table 1 Features of Atopic Dermatitis, Primary Irritant Dermatitis, and Infectious Dermatitis in the Newborn

	Atopic dermatitis	Primary irritant	Infectious dermatitis
Age of onset	Usually not before 3 months, rarely at end of first month, not at birth	Any time during first month	Any time
Family history	High incidence of respiratory allergy, hay fever, atopic dermatitis	None	May have bacterial carrier in family
Skin lesions	Weeping, vesicular, scaling; little lichenification before 4 months; extensor surfaces, cheeks, ears and scalp; symmetrical; rarely diaper area alone	Bright red, weeping; less scaling; any site may be involved but mostly diaper area, perianal area; may not be symmetrical	Weeping, much crusting; perioral, nasal, umbilical and diaper areas; punched out ulcers frequent on buttocks, perineum
Pruritis	Marked, precedes lesion	May be variable; follows lesions	Little
Culture	Often negative	Often negative	Positive-*Staphylococcus aureus*, *Streptococci*, *Enterococci*, *Candida albicans*, *Pseudomonas*
Other skin lesions	Associated "seborrheic" lesions ichthyosis vulgaris frequent; not seen until after 3 months of age	Usually none	Usually none; may be a complication of congenital defects; bullous lesions frequent
Consequence of delay in treatment	May improve spontaneously	Usually gets worse locally	Usually gets worse locally; satellite lesions develop nearby and at a distance
Incidence	Very rare	Very common	Common

Source: Ref. 1.

Histologically, these four stages are represented by (1) vasodilation (accompanied locally by the release of vasoactive substances including histamine, acetylcholine, kinins, serotonin, norepinephrine, prostoglandins, and others not yet chemically defined) and (2) infiltration of acute and chronic inflammatory cells into the epidermis. Edema of the Malpighian layer follows, which causes rupture of intercellular bridges, microvesicle formation (spongiosis), loss of epidermal integrity. Epidermal proliferation (3) and imperfect formation of a new stratum corneum, some cells of which may retain their nuclei (parakeratosis), can then be seen. This results in (4) thickening of the dermis and epidermis because of a downward proliferation of the rete ridges (acanthosis). The histologic features are comparable for all of the eczemas except when the infiltrate causing it is of a specific type (e.g., histiocytosis X).

It can be perceived from the preceding discussion that recognition of eczema is not difficult. But since its course and clinical picture may be quite variable, it is often difficult to distinguish different types of eczema from one another, and the histologic picture may not be helpful.

Although the causes of eczema in the adult comprise a formidable list, the causes of this disorder in the newborn are less numerous. Furthermore, the most common types of eczema in the adult are among the least common in the newborn. Indeed, eczema is a much less common disorder in the neonate than in an infant older than 2 months of age [1].

During the first months of life, the causes of eczema (Table 2) may be considered under two broad categories: exogenous and endogenous. The exogenous causes include primary irritant contact dermatitis, physical agents (light, cold, or heat), allergic eczematous contact dermatitis, and infection. The endogenous group may, for the purposes of discussion, be divided into those disorders in which the skin is predominantly involved and those in which the cutaneous eruption reflects serious systemic disease.

Irritating chemical substances, excessive washing, chafing, prolonged exposure to solar light, cold, and wind, and infection by bacteria and fungi more frequently cause eczematous eruptions during the neonatal period than allergy to food or topically applied agents.

CONTACT DERMATITIS

Two types of contact dermatitis may be distinguished (Table 2): primary irritant contact dermatitis, with nonspecific damage to the skin caused by the contactant; and allergic contact dermatitis, caused by specific hypersensitivity to the contactant. This paper will deal exclusively with primary irritant contact dermatitis.

Table 2 Causes of Eczema in the Newborn

Exogenous		With the cutaneous process predominant	Endogenous	
			With the cutaneous process predominant	Cutaneous process secondary to a systemic process[a]
Primary irritant		Infantile eczema, atopic seborrhea, "cradle cap"		Wiskott-Aldrich syndrome
Allergic	Contact dermatitis			Congenital sex-linked agammaglobulinemia
Bacteria				Leiner's disease with C dysfunction
Fungi	Infection	Desquamative erythroderma		Ataxia-telangiectasia
Light				Chronic granulomatous disease
				Phenylketonuria
Cold	Physical agents	Ritter's disease		Ahistidinemia
Heat		Congenital ichthyosiform erythroderma		Mucopolysaccharidoses
				Hartnup's disease
Allergic component	Insect bites			Acrodermatitis enteropathica
				Gluten-sensitive enteropathy
		"Diaper dermatitis"		Anhidrotic ectodermal dysplasia
				Histiocytosis X
				Long arm 18 deletion syndrome
				Hereditary acrokeratotic poikiloderma

[a]This list is not all-inclusive. Many additional reports exist of an eczematous process forming part of a syndrome.

Source: Ref. 1.

Primary irritant contact dermatitis (primary irritation) is an inflammatory response induced by a substance that disturbs the normal structure of the skin. No specific or allergic hypersensitivity to the substance is involved.

Pathogenesis

An irritant contact dermatitis will occur in all normal individuals if the contactant is of sufficient strength and if it acts upon the skin for a sufficiently long period of time. The amount of exposure required usually depends primarily on the innate destructive properties of the contactant and its concentration. Exposure to a potent irritant, such as a strong alkali, may induce intense inflammation within hours, while exposure to a mild irritant, such as a detergent, may require weeks to induce a dermatitis.

Although irritant contact dermatitis is not the result of specific hypersensitivity, certain individuals may be constitutionally more susceptible than others to the effects of irritants. The atopic individual is particularly susceptible to irritant contact dermatitis. Such patients have a lower threshold to itching and develop dermatitis more readily when exposed to detergents or wool.

The individual's constitutional predisposition and the nature of the contactant are the primary factors in inducing primary irritation. However, once the epidermis is damaged and the normal barrier function of the skin is lost, many factors may become involved in producing the subsequent inflammation. Damaged skin has increased susceptibility to many additional irritants, including minor irritants that have little effect upon intact skin. There frequently occurs, therefore, a "snowball" effect. Rubbing, scratching, and bacterial overgrowth may further contribute to and exacerbate the inflammation. The mechanism by which an irritant substance damages the skin depends upon its specific characteristics.

ETIOLOGY OF DIAPER RASH

Irritation of the diaper area plagues not only afflicted infants, but also their parents and physician. There are many recognized specific causes of diaper rash (monilial, contact, ammoniacal, or bacterial), but the diaper itself produces a unique environment that makes the skin of the perineum, buttocks, and thighs vulnerable to insult. Successful treatment and prevention of diaper rash not only requires attention to the specific etiologic agent but also to the environment of the diaper area.

Many believe that the time of the disposable diaper is at hand and the end of the diaper pail is near (here) [2]. Ten to 20 years from now, washable cloth diapers are as likely to be forgotten as the washable sanitary pads of 50 years ago. If disposable diapers still have faults, let us work to improve them for "they are here to stay."

Since 1877, when Parrott first described an eruption in the diaper area, repeated efforts have been made to find a single explanation for this affliction. Parrott described both a vesicular and papular form of the disorder and ascribed the latter to syphilis, calling it lenticular syphilis. The idea that syphilis was a major cause of diaper rashes persisted well into the early years of the twentieth century.

At the turn of the century, various efforts were being made to explain "diaper rash" on the basis of nutrition, alkalinity of feces, infection, and irritation, both chemical and mechanical. In 1915, Zahorsky [3] called attention to the almost constant association of the odor of ammonia in the diaper area with eruption in the diaper area. This association was not clarified, however, until Cooke [4,5] isolated *Brevibacterium ammoniagenes* and demonstrated its role in the production of ammonia in urine.

The clarification of the problem of ammoniacal dermatitis was important, but led, unfortunately, to overemphasis of this mechanism of diaper rash production to the exclusion of all other factors. In fact, until recently most textbooks of pediatrics mentioned only ammoniacal dermatitis under the heading "diaper rash." In 1961, Burgoon [6] and his associates first clearly stated that "diaper rash" is not a specific disorder but a reaction of the skin in a localized area. They pointed out that a variety of morphologic changes are produced by many causative factors. The authors divided these factors into predisposing and activating.

Another way of classifying diaper area eruptions is that of Koblenzer [2], who divided these disorders into three groups:

1. Those occurring whether diapers are worn or not
2. Those indicative of latent tendencies triggered by wearing diapers
3. Those occurring in nonpredisposed individuals as the direct consequence of wearing diapers

We are concerned here with the direct consequences of wearing diapers. The contribution of the diaper per se to rashes in the diaper area has been a point of contention for many years [7]. The diaper for babies in the early decades of this century consisted of cloth. The last was a wool overgarment similar in style and function to present day plastic pants. In the 1930s and 1940s rubber pants became popular but were available in large sizes only. The smaller baby wore diapers with or without woven pants, and was usually placed on a quilted pad. All of these techniques drew urine away from the baby's diaper area and allowed air to enter. During the 1950s the plastic pants in sizes suitable for infants under 3 months became popular. It is probably more than coincidence that monilial diaper rash was recognized as an important entity at that time. Burgoon and

Table 3 Frequency of Diaper Rash by Type of Rash and Kind of Diaper

		Miliaria	Pyoderma	Monilia	Other	Total rashes
Pampers	61	15	9	8	1	33
%		24.6	14.8	13.1	1.6	54.1
Cloth with plastic pants	61	8	2	5	5	20
%		13.1	3.3	8.2	8.2	32.8
Cloth alone	11	1	0	1	0	2
%		9.1	0	9.1	0	18.2
Miscellaneous	13	0	0	2	0	2
%		0	0	15.4	0	15.4
Total	146	24	11	16	6	57
%		16.4	7.5	11	4.1	39

Source: Ref. 7.

Wright [8] speculated on several predisposing and activating factors, including "maceration caused by continuous contact with a wet diaper and increased by the moist heat produced by an impervious rubber cover." Thus, the technologic advance of occluding the small baby's bottom with impervious rubber pants may have led to the considerable frequency of the monilial variety of diaper rash.

The convenience and watertight properties of the disposable plasticized paper diaper led to its widespread use and popularity. A recent report [7] has shown the frequency of diaper rash to be considerably increased in infants wearing disposable diapers as compared to cloth alone or cloth with plastic pants (Table 3).

Bare, healthy skin is smooth, shiny, and dry. Being separated by a fatty layer from the rest of the body, it is appreciably cooler than the interior, and its pH is lower. One cannot generalize, however, because, whereas the above statement may well be true of an area like the forearm, different conditions prevail in the axillae or more pertinently for the neonate, in the groins and gluteal cleft [1]. In these so-called intertriginous areas, the skin is warmer, moister, and, in certain areas, has a higher pH. Despite these regional differences, however, the skin of most individuals remains healthy and intact most of the time.

What happens when these areas are challenged by repeated exposure under occlusive cover? Wearing a diaper, especially when it lies within an occlusive cover, will produce a much warmer and more humid environment and thus even without the presence of urine or feces will materially affect the skin's defenses. Add to this the friction induced by movement, and the integrity of the skin in the diaper area may be compromised. Cases of direct irritant contact dermatitis constitute the vast majority of patients with diaper dermatitis.

A series of experiments were therfore conducted in our laboratory to discern the effects of occlusion on predisposing the skin to primary irritation.

Materials and Methods

Friction Device: The friction device utilized is as previously described [9]. Briefly, it consists of a variable speed, motor driven head or slider which recipro-cates in a 2-in. travel. The head can be covered with any test material. Three pairs of electric strain gauges are connected through a bridge amplifier to a strip recorder. One strain gauge pair measures the tension between the two feet ap-plied to the skin with adhesive. The adjustment of these feet is set to eliminate skin movement during testing. The second set of strain gauges reads spring ten-sion applied to the skin as normal load. Since there are small variations in skin surface, normal load readings are taken while the head is moving and an average load is used. Variation is kept within 5.0% by moving the instrument slightly until a smooth area is found. The third pair of strain gauges is mounted on the shaft of the friction head at right angles to the travel. This measures directly the frictional force exerted by the movement of the friction head. Static and kinetic friction can be determined from each recording. Calibration is accomplished by direct application of weights to the point of strain. The coefficient of friction, μ, is obtained from the following equation:

$$\mu = \frac{f}{F_N}$$

where F_N is the normal force of friction determined experimentally as described.

In Vivo Testing: Prior to testing, hair was removed from shins using commer-cially available thioglycolic acid. Testing was performed in a controlled environ-ment room at 22°C and 50% relative humidity. Hydration of the skin was pro-duced by occlusion of the whole lower legs with plastic wrap for 7 hr. Friction determinations were made immediately after removing wrapping.

Occlusive Chamber Irritation Assay: Webril pads (10 mm) contained in 12 mm aluminum chambers were moistened with 0.1 ml of the test solutions (tap water, distilled water, or 0.12% urea in distilled water) and applied to the volar surface of subjects' forearms. The chambers were taped in place using cloth Dermicel first aid tape and covered with stockinette bandage. Following a 24 hr exposure period, the chambers were removed and graded for erythema and hydration after a 30 min reaction period. The following grading system for both param-eters was utilized: ± = slight; 1 = definite but not over the entire area; 2 = defi-nite covering entire area.

For pretreatment experiments, a slight excess of zinc oxide paste was used and spread over the test site with a glass rod.

Results

Initially, experiments were conducted to determine the effects of occlusion alone on skin hydration and irritation. For this purpose, test sites were occluded with aluminum discs to simulate a diaper situation. The disc alone as well as the disc containing a Webril patch soaked with distilled water were employed.

As shown in Table 4, occlusion of the skin effected hydration of the test sites. Irritation was also observed in both cases but more severe where water was applied via the Webril patch. These results indicate that the hydration effect seen under occlusion may be largely from subcutaneous water and that penetration of surface water has less of an effect than expected. In contrast, erythema appeared to be more closely related to surface water as indicated by the higher scores on the sites where distilled water was applied.

Based on these observations, an additional experiment was conducted comparing the effects of distilled water with tap warer in terms of skin irritation and hydration upon occlusion. The results obtained are shown in Table 5 and indicate hydration and irritation with use of either. The data obtained indicated

Table 4 The Effects of Occlusion on Skin Hydration and Irritation[a]

	Hydration	Irritation
Occlusive disc alone	1.7	0.8
Occlusive disc with distilled water	1.7	2.1

[a]Results expressed as the ratio of the sum of the scores over the number of test sites.

Table 5 The Effects of Water Type on Skin Hydration and Irritation Due to Occlusion[a]

	Hydration	Irritation
Distilled water	1.7	2.1
Tap water	1.3	2.4

[a]Results expressed as the ratio of the sum of the scores divided by the number of test sites.

Table 6 Effects of Site Environment on Skin Hydration and
Irritation Due to Occlusion[a]

	Hydration	Irritation
Disc alone	1.9	0.8
Disc + dry pad	1.1	1.1
Disc + pad + distilled water	1.7	2.1
Disc + pad + tap water	1.3	2.4

[a]Results expressed as the ratio of the sum of the scores divided by the
 number of test sites.

greater skin hydration with distilled water while greater irritation was effected
with tap water. However, statistical significance was not achieved.

Table 6 shows a summary of the effects of site environment on skin hydration and irritation due to occlusion. As can be observed, skin hydration and
irritation were produced under all conditions. However, the greatest amount of
hydration observed was effected using the disc alone which again indicates the
importance of subcutaneous water in causing hydration by occlusion. In contrast, the greatest amount of irritation observed was produced by tap water, possibly showing the importance of surface irritants which penetrate the skin following hydration.

Subsequently, an additional experiment was performed investigating the possible effects of an irritant present in water applied to the skin using the Webril
patch. For this purpose, 0.12% urea was utilized (as a constituent of urine) and
compared with tap water and a distilled water control. Results are shown in
Table 7. Skin hydration and irritation were produced on occlusion at all test
sites. In terms of irritation, the urea solution effected erythema comparable to
that of tap water but somewhat more than the distilled water control. The data
again indicate a role of surface irritants in producing a reaction upon occlusion
but apparently not as would be expected. The irritation reactions produced by
occlusion alone are noteworthy.

In addition to the above studies, an experiment was performed to determine
if skin hydration and irritation due to occlusion could be prevented by some
pretreatment. Test skin sites were treated with zinc oxide paste prior to occlusion with the discs containing the Webril patch saturated with tap water. As
shown in Table 8, pretreatment of the test sites with zinc oxide paste prevented
virtually all occlusion-induced hydration and irritation. It would appear that
the paste used has the ability to somehow allow subcutaneous water through
but prevent that water from recontacting the skin to effect hydration and irritation.

Table 7 Effects of Irritant Solution on Skin Hydration and Irritation Due to Occlusion[a]

	Distilled water	Tap water	0.12% Urea
Irritation	2.1	2.4	2.4
Hydration	1.7	1.3	1.4

[a]Results expressed as the ratio of the sum of the scores divided by the number of test sites.

Table 8 Effects of Pretreatment on Skin Hydration and Irritation Due to Occlusion[a]

	Control[b]	Zinc oxide paste
Irritation	1.3	0.3
Hydration	1.0	0.0

[a]Webril pads saturated with 0.1 ml tap water.
[b]Results expressed as the ratio of the sum of the scores divided by the number of test sites.

Table 9 Effects of Pretreatment on Skin Hydration and Irritation Due to Occlusion[a]

	Control[b]	Zinc oxide paste
Irritation	1.0	0.27
Hydration	1.0	0.00

[a]Webril pads saturated with 0.12% urea in tap water.
[b]Results expressed as the ratio of the sum of the scores divided by the number of test sites.

Similarly, a study was performed using 0.12% urea in tap water as the irritant solution following pretreatment of the test sites with zinc oxide paste. As noted above, zinc oxide paste prevented development of hydration and irritation due to occlusion and with urea and tap water present. Although a successful prophylactic treatment, no mechanism of action for zinc oxide paste is known (Table 9).

In addition to examining the effects of occlusion on skin hydration and irritation, a series of experiments was conducted to determine the effects of occlu-

Table 10 Effects of Hydration on Coefficients of Friction in Vivo[a]

$\mu \pm$ SE:	0.33 ± 0.02	0.86 ± 0.08
Range:	$0.21 - 0.63$	$0.60 - 1.80$
N:	15	15

[a]Nonwoven pulp fabric used on friction slider.

Table 11 Effects of Lubricants on Skin Friction in Vivo

		% change in friction	
Treatment	Dry[a]	Dry[b]	Hydrated[b]
Silicone oil[c]	−55.0	+3.0	−23.4
Petroleum jelly	−69.0	−36.0	−90.0

[a]Polyethylene film used on friction slider.
[b]Nonwoven pulp fabric used on friction slider.
[c]Dow Corning 472 fluid, glycol polysiloxane.

sion on friction between a diaper liner and skin. Friction induced by movement may further compromise the integrity of the skin in the diaper area. For this purpose, a friction machine was used as described above and the slider was covered with nonwoven fabric to simulate a diaper liner. Friction determinations were made on both dry and hydrated skin in vivo.

As can be observed in Table 10, hydration of the skin significantly increased the coefficient of friction between fabric and skin. This supports the hypothesis that friction between the diaper and hydrated skin assists in deterioration of the integument's integrity.

Further, similar friction determinations were made in vivo following application of two popular lubricant materials to determine if such pretreatment may help alleviate frictional effects on dry and hydrated skin in a diaper. Silicone oil and petroleum jelly were utilized and applied just prior to measurement of the frictional coefficient. Results are shown in Table 11. As can be observed, lubricants can have varying effects on friction depending upon the nature of the contacting surfaces. For example, silicone oil appears to serve as a lubricant between polyethylene film and skin but not between fabric and skin. In contrast, petroleum jelly lubricated in both situations. Noteworthy is the difference in effect of the lubricants when applied on either dry or hydrated skin. On hydrated skin both silicone oil and petroleum jelly provided substantial lubricating action with the latter providing the greatest effect. These results tend to support the use of lubricating materials in the diaper area to help prevent skin maceration.

Discussion

As previously stated, the individual's constitutional predisposition and the nature of the contactant are the main factors in inducing primary irritation. However, once the epidermis is damaged and the normal barrier function of the skin is lost, many factors may be involved in producing inflammation. Damaged skin has increased susceptibility to many additional irritants, including minor irritants that have little effect upon intact skin. We are concerned here with the direct consequences of wearing diapers, a predisposing factor at least in irritation in the area of the diaper.

The question most frequently raised is: what happens when these areas are challenged by repeated exposure under occlusion to irritant materials? Wearing a diaper produces a warmer more humid environment and thus, even without the presence of urine or feces, may materially affect the skin's defenses. Add to this the friction induced by movement, and the integrity of the skin in the diaper area may be compromised.

The results obtained demonstrated the effects of occlusion on skin. Occlusion effected skin hydration whether external water was applied to the test sites or not. In fact, the greatest amount of hydration was noted where the aluminum disc was used without a Webril patch or water. These findings indicate that the hydration effect seen under occlusion may be largely from subcutaneous water and that penetration of surface water has less of an effect than expected.

In contrast, erythema appeared to be more closely related to surface water, since tap water effected erythema comparable to that of an urea solution but higher than the distilled water control.

A series of experiments was also performed to determine the effects of occlusion on friction as between a diaper liner and skin. The results obtained support the hypothesis that friction between the diaper and hydrated skin assists in deteriorating the integrity of the integument.

A series of experiments was performed to determine if hydration and irritation due to occlusion could be prevented or treated. Pretreatment of the test sites with zinc oxide paste was used because of its frequent utilization. The results clearly demonstrated the ability of the paste virtually to eliminate hydration and irritation due to occlusion. Apparently, the zinc oxide has the ability to allow subcutaneous water through while preventing contact of surfact water and irritants.

A study was conducted in attempt to determine if friction between diaper and skin could be decreased to help prevent maceration due primarily to the environment. Two treatments were employed and both successfully reduced friction between hydrated skin and fabric. These results serve to support the use of materials intended to reduce hydration and friction in the diaper area.

The results obtained demonstrate that the diaper area environment can serve as a predisposing factor in diaper dermatitis. Occlusion alone can effect hydration and irritation and assist in the deterioration of the integument in the diaper region. Consequently, successful treatment and prevention of diaper rash not only requires attention to a specific etiologic agent but also to the environment of the diaper area.

REFERENCES

1. Solomon LM, Esterly NB: Eczema, in *Neonatal Dermatology*. Saunders, Philadelphia, 1973.
2. Koblenzer PJ: Diaper dermatitis—an overview. Clin Pediatr 12:386-392, 1973.
3. Zahorsky J: The ammoniacal diaper in infants and young children. Am J Dis Child 10:436, 1915.
4. Cooke JV: The etiology and treatment of ammonia dermatitis of the gluteal region of infants. Am J Dis Child 22:481, 1921.
5. Cooke JV: Dermatitis of the diaper region in infants. Arch Dermatol Syph 14:539, 1926.
6. Burgoon CJ, Urbach F, Grover WD: Diaper dermatitis. Pediatr Clin North Am 18:835, 1961.
7. Wiener F: The relationship of diapers to diaper rashes in the one-month-old infant. J Pediat 95:422, 1979.
8. Burgoon C, Wright C: Diaper dermatitis, in *Nelson's Textbook of Pediatrics*. Saunders, Philadelphia, 1964.
9. McCormack JJ, Fisher LB, Boisits EK: Human skin and friction: A clear appraisal. Presented at the Annual Meeting of the Society of Cosmetic Chemists, New York City, December 1, 1978.

15

Factors Influencing Infant Diaper Dermatitis

WILLIAM E. JORDAN and TED L. BLANEY
The Procter and Gamble Company, Cincinnati, Ohio

Few infants emerge from their diaper-wearing years (birth to approximately 3 or more years of age) without experiencing one or more episodes of dermatitis of the diapered area, customarily described as diaper rash. Parrott first described eruptions in the diaper area in 1877, although, as Burgoon et al. [1] point out, "it seems reasonable to assume that a covering to catch the drippings of the socially inept infant antedate this observation," hence, one can also assume that diaper dermatitis was evident earlier. In 1915 Zahorsky [2] noted the frequency with which diaper area eruptions were associated with the ammoniacal diaper. In 1921, Cooke [3] established the source of this ammonia as the product of bacterial degradation of urine. This resulted in a single-minded focus on ammonia as the sole cause of eruptions of the diaper area until 1961, when Burgoon and his co-workers noted that diaper dermatitis, or diaper rash, is not a single entity but a variety of morphologic responses of the skin to multiple causative factors which they classified as either "predisposing" (genetically inherited traits or systemic disease altering response of the cutaneous system), or "activating" (those factors which may initiate dermatitis in the predisposed infant). Koblenzer [4] subsequently classified diaper area eruptions into three groups:

1. Those occurring whether or not diapers are worn. These were described as rare and mainly result from systemic disease.
2. Those indicative of latent tendencies triggered by wearing diapers. These

were described as the result of hyperreactive skin and/or seborrheic dermatitis and, according to Koblenzer, make up the bulk of "recidivist" cases of diaper dermatitis.

3. Those occurring in nonpredisposed individuals as a direct consequence of wearing diapers. Koblenzer recognized two types: allergic contact dermatitis and direct irritant contact dermatitis.

Koblenzer states that allergic contact dermatitis is relatively rare, while irritant contact dermatitis constitutes the vast majority of patients with diaper dermatitis. He places "tidemark" dermatitis, ammoniacal dermatitis, and fecal contact dermatitis in the latter category, and infections with yeast, bacteria, and/or viruses may complicate any of the conditions described.

Koblenzer's categories 1 and 2 reflect the "predisposing" factors of Burgoon et al., and category 3 those characterized as "activating." This classification places perspective on the potential role of the diaper in diaper rash.

This section will deal only with nonsystemic factors that may influence the development of diaper rash. Our analysis suggests that these factors include the kind of diaper, age, diaper change frequency, and diaper area care practices.

POTENTIAL EFFECTS ATTRIBUTED TO THE DIAPER

As Koblenzer noted, skin rashes of the infant's perineal area may occur in the absence of a diaper, but those rashes of most frequent concern to physicians and parents are associated with its use. Kahn [5] described the most common cause of diaper dermatitis as a variety of irritant materials held in intimate contact with the skin by diapers and rubber or plastic pants. Altchek [6] holds a similar view:

Diaper rash is set off by moisture, heat, and soiling. The main factors are infrequent changes and the use of plastic, waterproof outer diaper covers. The latter keeps the outer clothes and mother dry but acts like a heat shield and will cause damaging high temperature and humidity in the involved area. The skin develops erythema, edema, vesicles, weeping, and secondary bacterial and Candidal infection.

Thus, the diaper is assigned a prominent role in onset of diaper rash.

In the United States, two general types of infant diapers are commonly used: reusable cotton cloth and single-use (disposable). Each is produced by a number of manufacturers.

Cotton cloth diapers are made as either a single-layered "birdseye" or a double-layered "gauze" diaper. Most reusable diapers are rectangular in shape and designed for folding to fit a wide range of infant sizes and ages. A more or less "hour-glass-shaped" cloth diaper, contoured to fit the infant better, is also available. It is common practice to employ double and triple cloth diapers to provide adequate moisture-absorption capacity, particularly for infants voiding large quantities of urine.

In the United States, most users of cloth diapers (about 90%) [7] employ rubber or plastic overpants with a frequency ranging from constant to "only at nap-time." These overpants most commonly have elastic legbands, to minimize leakage from wetted diapers, and snaps, elastic waistbands, or "hook-and-loop" fasteners for fitting over the diaper.

It is clear from the statements of Kahn and Altchek that medical opinion argues against the use of plastic or rubber overpants with cloth diapers. The high frequency of use of overpants emphasizes the importance that most mothers attach to the ability of a diapering system to "contain" well, and protect the infant's clothing, bedclothing, furniture and, quite possibly, her own mental and physical well-being.

In the United States, the single-use, or disposable, diaper has been available for many years. Within the last 10 years, since the unitized panty diaper displaced the "insert," the disposable diaper has become the choice of a majority of mothers.

Disposable diapers are available in a variety of sizes, varying in dimension and absorption capacity, to accommodate the needs of infants ranging from premature to 3½ years or older. Most disposable diapers sold today consist of an absorbent core made from fluffed highly purified cellulose pulp, a plastic outer cover, or backsheet, and a nonwoven fabric liner, which contacts the infant's skin. The liner is designed to promote passage of urine through to the absorptive core while keeping a dry surface next to the infant's skin. However, the integral plastic backsheet has been the cause for concern regarding the "breathability" of the diaper, attracting the same criticism levelled at the plastic or rubber overpants utilized with cloth diapers, i.e., that they are "air- and water-tight," hence occlusive to an unacceptable degree. It is a common misconception that the "containment" effectiveness of disposable diapers derives from their "sealing" against the skin at potential points of leakage, e.g., the legs and waist. This is not the case; containment is mainly a matter of design in the placement of the absorptive material making up the core and the use of liner fabrics that permit the rapid penetration and dispersion of urine into the core material.

Clinical and Experimental Studies

The studies reported here have been designed to determine the potential effects on diaper rash incidence and severity resulting from a choice of cloth or disposable diapers. Clinical studies comparing cloth diapers to disposable diapers are discussed, as well as experimental studies on the effects of occlusivity on skin bacterial growth and the effects of diaper occlusivity on skin temperature.

The comparative effects on incidence and/or severity of diaper rash of using disposable diapers and cloth diapers with varying degrees of occlusivity have been studied in the United States and in Japan. Cloth diapers are used in the United States in conjunction with plastic or rubber overpants designed and used so as to be at least as occlusive as disposable diapers. In Japan, cloth diapers are used mainly in conjunction with woven synthetic fabric water-repellent overpants that, by virtue of their inherent porosity, are considered to be less occlusive than either disposable diapers or cloth diapers as they are used in the United States.

Infants aged 3-24 months were studied. Irritation of the skin of the diaper area was evaluated by investigators unaware of product identity using a scale of 0-4, with 0 indicating freedom from rash and 4 severe eruption. Four regions of the skin covered by the diaper were examined separately: waistband, genitals, buttocks, and legs (thighs). Severity of lesions and the total area of the skin affected were both considered in determining a grade. Skin redness (erythema), rash (papules, pustules, edema), and skin integrity (ulceration, scaling) were the morphologic features to which attention was directed; no attempt was made to assign a specific etiology to the rash. An overall grade was assigned after each of the four regions was evaluated and was weighted towards the rash grade of the region with most severe lesions. Details of study designs are contained in the Appendix.

Table 1 summarizes the results of these studies, two in the United States and two in Japan. These results indicate that, as typically used, disposable diapers and cloth diapers do not differ in their influence on diaper rash. Further, cloth diapers used with minimally occlusive overpants do not appear to differ from those used with overpants of relatively high occlusivity in their influence on diaper rash, since both are equivalent to disposable diapers. However, this equivalence cannot be taken to indicate that occlusion is of no consequence; rather, it might suggest that a majority of mothers change diapers with acceptable frequency, or that the diaper is less occlusive than assumed.

Experimental evidence is available on the effects of occlusion of the skin. Marples [8] reported that the application of moisture-proof films directly to the skin for 24 hrs results in a sharp rise in the microbial population of the occluded area, presumably due to accumulation of transpired skin moisture and favorable skin temperature.

We have observed that these effects may be modified when a moisture-absorbent material is interposed between the skin and the occluding film. In this study, the skin of young adults was occluded with moisture-proof film, under which absorbent diaper core material was placed prior to sealing the film to the skin, and film under which the absorbent core material was moistened with four

Table 1 Comparative Effects of Disposable and Cloth Diaper Use on Diaper Rash

Study location	Season	Diaper used	No. of infants	None–slight	Slight–moderate	Moderate–severe	Diaper rash score[b]	LSD$_{95}$[c]
				No. of infants with rash rated[a]				
United States	Summer	Cloth	70	31	37	2	0.67	0.17
		Disposable	77	33	43	1	0.73	
United States	Winter	Cloth	83	49	34	0	0.89	0.14
		Disposable	80	55	23	2	0.87	
Japan	Fall	Cloth	75	48	22	5	1.01	0.21
		Disposable	75	44	25	6	1.18	
Japan	Spring	Cloth	85	67	18	0	0.79	0.17
		Disposable	84	69	13	2	0.77	

[a]None to slight rash = < 1.0; slight to moderate rash = ≥ 1.0 < 2.5; moderate to severe rash = ≥ 2.5.

[b]Based on the evaluation technique described in the Appendix. 0 = No evidence of rash; 1 = slight rash (detectable erythema); 2 = mild rash (moderate to severe erythema and/or scaling, slight edema, and papules); 3 = moderate rash (moderate to severe erythema and scaling, slight to moderate ulceration, moderate to severe papules and edema); 4 = severe rash (severe ulceration, papules, edema, erythema).

[c]Least significant difference, 95% level of confidence.

209

Table 2 Modification of the Effects of Occlusion of the Skin

Treatment	Period of occlusion (hr)	Mean bacterial count/cm^2
Skin unoccluded (control)	—	1×10^3
Skin occluded with film only	24	2.1×10^6
Skin occluded with film, plus dry cellulose pulp	24	8×10^1
Skin occluded with film, plus cellulose pulp to which 4X by weight distilled water was added	4	1.2×10^2
	7	1×10^3
	24	3.6×10^5

times its weight of distilled water. The skin flora was subsequently assayed by the technique of Williamson [9] at various times up to 24 hrs after the occluding films were applied.

The results, summarized in Table 2, suggest that a *dry* diaper, even under an occlusive film, does not provide environmental conditions conducive to bacterial growth on the infant skin. However, the data suggest that a wet diaper can provide sufficient moisture to promote bacterial growth, if left on the infant for a sufficient period of time. Fecal matter present in the diaper may also have its own effects on the skin as well as providing a dramatically heavier inoculum of bacteria for urine that may already be present, as can inadequately washed cloth diapers.

We have further investigated the "hot house" effect attributed to disposable diapers by determining the skin temperature within the diapered area and comparing it with that of undiapered areas of the skin. A rapid response thermistor skin temperature probe and a thermistor thermometer were used to determine skin temperature at several points within the diapered area and two points not normally covered. Table 3 summarizes the results.

These data show that the temperature of the diaper-covered areas does not differ markedly from that of adjacent undiapered areas. The temperature of the buttocks' skin, for example, is not greatly different from that of the outer aspect of the thigh, and the pubic and intertriginous areas have temperatures quite similar to that of the abdomen. There is, clearly, no "hot-house" effect apparent.

Overall, the data lead to the conclusion that the occlusive, or "air- and water-tight," properties of the disposable diaper have been everestimated. In a properly sized and fitted diaper, there is ample air circulation through the waist and leg openings by the bellows action of the diaper that accompanies the movements of the normal healthy infant.

Table 3 Skin Temperature Within the Diapered Area
(Disposable Diaper)

Site	Skin temperature (°F)	
	Mean[a]	SD
Diapered area		
Pubic	95.3	0.3
Intertriginous	97.9	0.3
Buttocks	89.4	0.8
Normally exposed skin		
Abdomen	95.5	0.2
Outer aspect of thigh	90.6	0.4

[a]Study base = 25 infants.

Age

Considering the changes in diet, physiological state, and environmental insult
that the infant undergoes in the first months of life, it would not be surprising
if diaper rash incidence and severity change to some degree with age. A retrospec-
tive study by Grant et al. [10] reported peak incidence of diaper rash among infants in the 7-9 months age range. In a study limited to 1-month-old infants,
Wiener [11] reported an extraordinary incidence and severity of diaper rash
(54%), one-third of which was severe, among those wearing disposable diapers.
This suggests the possibility that the 4-week-old group may be more prone to
diaper rash.

Our results support the findings of Grant et al. and disagree with those of
Wiener. Figure 1 illustrates the incidence and severity of diaper rash as reflected
by diaper rash score observed at various infant ages during one of our studies.
A slight peak in diaper rash among infants wearing either cloth or disposable
diapers is observed in the 6-10 months age range, decreasing thereafter. We also
conducted a detailed study concentrating on infants, ranging in age from newborn to 5 weeks at the beginning of the study, when they were assigned use of
disposable diapers. They were evaluated for diaper rash 3-4 weeks later, and at
biweekly intervals thereafter for 6 additional weeks. Figure 2 and Table 4 summarize these findings. Slight to moderate rash, graded as equal to or greater than
1.0 and less than 2.5, was observed in about one-third of the 212 infants at any
given time. Severe rash, graded as equal to or greater than 2.5, was detected in
1-4% of the infants, depending upon the examination period. The overall diaper

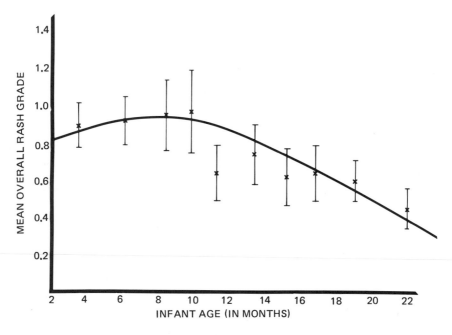

Figure 1 Diaper rash as a function of infant age.

rash score was 0.46 for all infants. There is no evidence of extraordinary rash among any of these very young infants, including the 1-month-old group.

Variability in the severity of rash is illustrated in Table 4. Few infants seemed consistently to maintain a significant level of diaper rash throughout the study period; more often it appeared relatively transient. In part, this may reflect specific actions taken by the mother, i.e., increased attention to diaper area care practices when she perceives her infant developing an unacceptable level of diaper rash.

Change Frequency

Prompt changing of the infant's soiled diaper (change frequency) is unanimously regarded as important in the control of diaper rash. Prolonged exposure of the skin to moisture can induce maceration, thus enhancing the susceptibility of the skin to irritant effects, and it is clearly desirable to minimize the duration of skin exposure to irritant materials that may be present in urine or fecal matter. However, our experience is that the ideal of changing the diaper immediately following each wetting or soiling is rarely met.

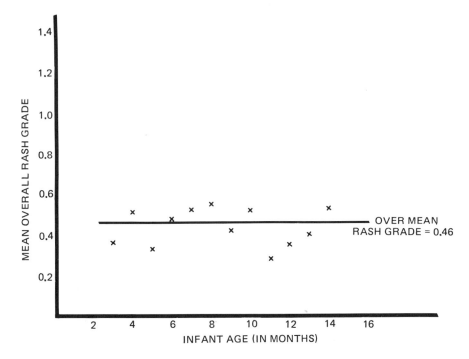

Figure 2 Diaper rash as a function of age among very young infants.

Newborns urinate more than 20 times daily, although this frequency drops markedly as the infant grows older, averaging 6.5 times at 1 year and older [12]. The frequency of diaper change observed seldom approaches these figures. In our most recent Market Research survey [7], the infant care habits of almost 1300 mothers of healthy infants ranging in age from newborn to 36 months of age were evaluated. This survey, summarized in Table 5, show that, overall, disposable diapers are changed with a slightly lower frequency, 5.05 times per day, than cloth, 5.30 changes per day, corresponding to a difference in wearing time of 13 min.

Age of the infant is an important variable; newborns are changed with a significantly higher frequency than older infants. Overall, there is, as expected, a pattern of decreasing change frequency of both cloth and disposable diapers as the infant grows older which, interestingly, coincides with decreasing diaper rash (Fig. 1). The infant voids less frequently but in greater volume. This imposes a requirement for greater absorbency on the diaper, which is met by increasing the quantity of absorbent material in disposables and by double and triple diapering with cloth diapers.

Table 4 Occurrence and Variability of Diaper Rash Among Very Young Infants[a] Wearing Disposable Diapers

Study period	% of Infants with rash score rated[b]	
	Slight-moderate	Moderate-severe
Occurrence		
Initial examination (after 3 or 4 weeks diaper use)	33	2
Second examination (2 weeks later)	34	4
Third examination (4 weeks later)	34	4
Fourth examination (6 weeks later)	33	2
Variability		
Rash detected once in 4 examinations	24	3.8
Rash detected twice in 4 examinations	22	1.4
Rash detected three times in 4 examinations	15	1.9
Rash detected four times in 4 examinations	6	0

[a]212 infants, ages 3-9 weeks at first examination. Product use (disposable diapers) begun at birth to 5 weeks of age.

[b]Based on evaluation technique described in the Appendix. Slight to moderate rash = $\geq 1.0 < 2.5$; moderate to severe rash = ≥ 2.5.

Table 6 summarizes data on change frequency, compiled from mothers' diary records, derived from another diaper rash study. As expected, change frequency is lower with older infants, although extremes in change frequency are evident in virtually every age range. There is good agreement between these diary data from a single study compared with the overall summary described in Table 5.

We have studied correlations between diaper change frequency and diaper rash, anticipating that increased change frequency would result in lower diaper rash frequency and/or severity. Within the normal change frequency range of mothers of infants in these studies, we have not found the correlation with diaper rash to be statistically significant.

The wide variation in change frequency observed in these tests might reflect a similar variation in the toilet habits of the infants, i.e., frequency of urination and defecation, and that mothers adjust their diapering frequency to those habits

Table 5 Diaper Change Frequency: Normal Infants

Age range (months)	Changes per day	
	Disposables	Cloth
0-3	7.6	7.76
4-6	6.37	8.05
7-9	6.95	7.22
10-12	6.53	7.49
13-15	5.87	5.82
16-18	5.42	5.58
19-21	5.14	5.21
22-24	4.22	4.18
25-27	3.33	4.49
28-30	2.69	2.39
31-33	1.97	2.45
34-36	1.82	1.31

[a]1395 mothers of diaper-wearing infants surveyed, with 1291 providing diary data. Overall change frequency 5.05/day for disposables, 5.30/day for cloth.

Source: Ref. 7.

as well as their own convenience. They do not knowingly allow the infant to remain in a soiled diaper for an extended time. We believe that any effects of diaper change frequency would be apparent only in a study requiring mothers to use specified change frequencies, e.g., three or four per day versus another group required to change perhaps six or eight times daily.

Diaper Area Care Practices

Those caring for infants are offered a variety of products and recommendations for the prevention or therapy of diaper rash. A wide variety of infant care products, powders, lotions, oils, ointments, creams, dietary supplements, and diaper laundry treatments are available, all potentially helpful in solving the problem of diaper rash. These preparations' mechanisms of action may include moisture absorbency, reducing mechanical trauma due to skin friction, barriers to prevent the macerating effects of moisture on the skin, and/or limiting the production of ammonia from urine by inhibition of growth of ammoniagenic bacteria. Dietary supplements reportedly modify the pH of urine to minimize or prevent skin irritation by the wet diaper.

Table 6 Diaper Change Frequency Among Infants 3-18 Months Old

Age range	No. of infants[a]	Change frequency			Diaper rash grade[b]	
		Mean	SD	Extremes	Mean	SD
3-6	29	6.6	1.2	4.6-9.8	1.30	0.72
7-9	49	6.9	1.6	4.0-10.5	1.23	0.57
10-12	96	6.5	1.5	3.8-10.5	1.13	0.57
13-15	115	6.2	1.6	3.0-9.9	1.1	0.50
16-18	63	5.7	1.0	3.3-8.7	1.07	0.45

[a]Data collected on 352 infants, all diapered in disposable diapers. Mothers kept diaries for 2 weeks. Rash levels were evaluated after 2 weeks.

[b]Based on the evaluation technique described in the Appendix. 0 = No evidence of rash; 1 = slight rash (detectable erythema); 2 = mild rash (moderate to severe erythema and/or scaling, slight edema, and papules); 3 = moderate rash (moderate to severe erythema and scaling, slight to moderate ulceration, moderate to severe papules and edema); 4 = severe rash (severe ulceration, papules, edema, erythema).

Effectiveness of these preparations may be uncertain in any given diaper rash episode because of the multiplicity of factors that may contribute to the development of diaper rash. Treatments whose action is predicated on a single cause of diaper rash will have limited prophylactic or therapeutic value.

To some extent, superficial infections of the skin of the diaper area may be regarded as complications of diaper rash initiated by irritant or allergic contact dermatitis, or other rashes which Koblenzer categorizes as 1 or 2. These infections will usually respond to specific therapy. Allergic or irritant contact dermatitis, once manifested, may also require specific therapies. However, their prevention seem more productive.

In the diaper area, prevention of contact between the skin and irritant or allergic materials is most readily accomplished by interposing a barrier cream or ointment between the skin and the insulting agent. Prompt removal of the insulting agent from the skin may also be effective and is best accomplished by use of soap and water, although a fine line must be drawn between thorough cleansing and overenthusiastic application that may itself result in defatting and irritating the skin, and hence predispose to the effects of irritants and/or allergens one is attempting to remove.

We have studied the effects of hygiene measures and the use of skin barrier preparations on the incidence and severity of diaper rash. Approximately equal numbers of mothers of 403 infants, aged 3-18 months, were directed to use one of six care regimens for 2 weeks following 2 weeks of undirected use of a control disposable diaper. The test regimens were as follows:

1. Daily bathing of the infant and use of soap and water to cleanse the diaper area at each diaper change. No diaper area care aids were employed.
2. Twice-weekly bathing of the infant and minimal cleansing of the diaper area at each change, preferably with tissue or the diaper itself. No diaper area care aids were employed.
3. The intensive cleansing procedures described in (1) and use of U.S.P. petrolatum at each change.
4. The infrequent cleansing procedures described in (2) and use of U.S.P. petrolatum at each change.
5. The intensive cleansing procedures described in (1) and use of a zinc oxide-based ointment at each change.
6. The infrequent cleansing procedures described in (2) and use of a zinc oxide-based ointment at each change.

The infants were examined and their rash levels evaluated before use of the test regimens and after 1 and 2 weeks of their employment by the mothers. Compliance with the study regimen was encouraged by asking mothers to keep a complete record of every diaper change and to contact the investigator if they became concerned or found it necessary to modify the procedure requested, and assuring them that no penalty would be incurred. Noncompliance was minimal, less than 2%.

Results are summarized in Table 7. The use of the zinc oxide-based ointment, with either of the more or less intensive cleansing procedures, resulted in a slightly and statistically significant lower diaper rash among infants in those test groups. In the absence of use of any barrier preparation, the more intensive cleansing procedure resulted in a slightly lower rash (statistically significant) than in the group employing the less intensive cleansing procedures. Curiously, petrolatum appeared to unfavorably affect the improvement otherwise observed with employment of the intensive cleansing procedure alone.

SUMMARY

We have attempted to define the role of selected factors, which we term "non-systemic," in diaper rash incidence and/or severity.

No differences were observed in the effects on diaper rash of the two diapering systems, disposables and cloth combined with plastic pants, in wide use in the United States. A comparison of a nominally less occlusive cloth diaper system, in which fabric overpants are used, with disposable diapers also failed to show different effects on diaper rash. We do not discount the potential effects of occlusion on the infant skin, but it appears that the normal wearing times of diapers are sufficiently short to prevent their manifestation, or that the occlusive properties of diapers are overestimated.

Table 7 Effects of Hygiene Measures and Skin Barrier Preparations on Diaper Rash

| Treatment | | | No. of infants with rash rated[b] | | |
Skin barrier preparation	Hygiene measures	Mean diaper[a] rash score	None–slight	Slight–moderate	Moderate–severe
None	Daily bathing, soap and water cleansing after each change	1.18[c] ⎤ LSD₉₅	25	49	0
	Twice weekly bathing, minimal cleansing after each change	1.25 ⎦ .07	9	59	0
U.S.P. petrolatum	Daily bathing, soap and water cleansing after each change	1.26 ⎤ LSD₉₅	16	53	0
	Twice weekly bathing, minimal cleansing after each change	1.21 ⎦ .07	14	44	1
Zinc oxide ointment	Daily bathing, soap and water cleansing after each change	1.06[c] ⎤ LSD₉₅	41	23	4
	Twice weekly bathing, minimal cleansing after each change	1.00[c] ⎦ .07	32	33	0

LSD₉₅ .09

[a] Based on the evaluation technique described in the Appendix. 0 = No evidence of rash; 1 = slight rash (detectable erythema); 2 = mild rash (moderate to severe erythema and/or scaling, slight edema, and papules); 3 = moderate rash (moderate to severe erythema and scaling, slight to moderate ulceration, moderate to severe papules and edema); 4 = severe rash (severe ulceration, papules, edema, and erythema).

[b] None to slight = < 1.0; slight to moderate = $\geqslant 1.0 < 2.5$; moderate to severe = > 2.5.

[c] Significantly different at the 95% confidence level.

Age is a factor in incidence and severity of diaper rash, with an apparent peak in the 6-10 months age range. Overall incidence and severity is not disturbing, even at young ages (<3 months), and decreases beyond 10 months.

These studies detected no correlation between diaper change frequency and diaper rash incidence and/or severity. However, mothers participating in these studies were permitted to maintain their normal change frequency, and it may be that these are adjusted by the mother to coincide with her infant's toilet habits and her own convenience.

Diaper area care practices were found to influence diaper rash incidence and severity, as measured by the techniques described. Increased bathing frequency and the use of a zinc oxide-based ointment were effective in reducing the incidence and severity of diaper rash by a statistically significant degree.

APPENDIX

Subject Selection

Infants were selected for participation in these tests on the basis of age (generally 3-24 months, with noted exceptions) and state of health, i.e., only "well" babies were included; those with systemic disease were excluded. Informed consent was secured from the parents or guardians of all infants and, where participants failed to complete the study, the mothers were questioned to assure that their withdrawal was unrelated to effects of test products.

Evaluation of Diaper Area Irritation

Irritation of the skin of the diaper area was evaluated on a scale of 0-4, with 0 indicating freedom from rash and 4 indicating a severe case. Four regions of the diaper area were examined: waistband, genitals, buttocks, and legs (thighs). Both severity of lesions and total area of the skin affected were considered. Skin redness (erythema), rash (papules, pustules, edema), and skin integrity (ulceration, scaling) were the morphologic features to which attention was directed. A photographic scale was also used as an aid in judging their type and intensity. No attempt was made to assign a specific etiology to the rash.

The same trained investigators separately made the observations and assigned a grade to each infant in any given study to ensure consistency of grading. All infants were presented for grading in a disposable diaper loosely fitted, hence the investigators were effectively "blinded" to the identity of the product actually being used. Following the evaluation of the diaper area, the mother replaced the disposable diaper with the assigned product. Proper lighting was provided using 3200°K for skin redness grading.

Test Design and Analysis

Our diaper rash tests were designed for covariant analysis, chosen because of the wide difference in frequency and severity of rash between babies. The covariant analysis is more sensitive to determining significant differences between treatments under these circumstances.

Generally, all infants were graded for diaper rash following a control period, followed by random assignment of the infants to a test group for 4 to 6 weeks. Skin grading period were generally two weeks apart. A typical test is outlined below.

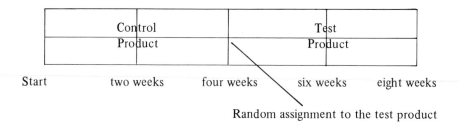

Control	Test
Product	Product

Start   two weeks   four weeks   six weeks   eight weeks

Random assignment to the test product

It has been our experience that most diaper rash uncomplicated by infection clears within a week of its peak. The 2 weeks between gradings allow for resolution of most previous episodes of diaper rash within a test group.

Unless otherwise specified by the study protocol, there were at least four grading periods, two during the control period and two or more during the test period. At each grading period, there were grades for four diaper area regions: waist, genital, buttocks, and legs, and an overall grade subjectively weighted toward the most severe rash present in any region rather than the average grade of the four regions.

Covariant analysis was performed for each region grade, the overall grade and the average rash grade, using the mean of the control period scores and the test period scores. All assumptions of covariant analysis were tested and fulfilled.

REFERENCES

1. Burgoon CJ, Urbach F, Glover, WD: Diaper dermatitis. Pediatr Clin North Am 18:835, 1961.
2. Zahorsky J: The ammoniacal diaper in infants and young children. Am J Dis Child 10:436, 1915.
3. Cooke JV: The etiology and treatment of ammonia dermatitis of the gluteal region of infants. Am J Dis Child 22:481, 1921.
4. Koblenzer PJ: Diaper dermatitis—an overview. Clin Pediatr 12:386, 1973.

5. Kahn G: Eczematoid eruptions in children. Pediatr Clin North Am 22:203, 1975.
6. Altchek A: Pediatric vulvovaginitis. Pediatr Clin North Am 19:559, 1972.
7. Procter & Gamble Company: Market Research Survey—1975.
8. Marples RR: The effect of hydration on the bacterial flora of the skin, in *Skin Bacteria and Their Role in Infection*, edited by Maibach HI, Hildick-Smith G. McGraw-Hill, New York, 1965.
9. Williamson P: Quantitative estimation of cutaneous bacteria, in *Skin Bacteria and Their Role in Infection*, edited by Maibach HI, Hildick-Smith G. McGraw-Hill, New York, 1965.
10. Grant WW, Street L, Fearnow RG: Diaper rashes in infancy. Clin Pediatr 12:714, 1973.
11. Wiener F: The relationship of diapers to diaper rashes in the one-month-old infant. J Pediatr 95:422, 1979.
12. Plenert U: Hiene VEB Verlag Volk U. Gesundheit/Berlin, 1966.

16

Contact Sensitization in Neonates and Infants

ERNST EPSTEIN

University of California Medical Center, San Francisco, California

INDUCTION OF DELAYED-TYPE CONTACT SENSITIVITY

Neonates can be sensitized to potent allergens, although not as easily as older children and adults [1-3].

Strauss [1] used a crude extract of *Rhus toxicodendron radicans* (poison ivy) to sensitize 35 of 48 newborns 1-4 days old. The crude extract ("ivy paste") was applied to the skin of the back and covered with glazed paper affixed with tape for 6-8 days. In some subjects an additional patch was applied to abraded skin; these infants were also fed an ivy extract while in the hospital. The sensitization test sites were negative at the time of test removal 6-8 days later.

Challenge patch testing was performed 2-4 weeks after the sensitization procedure using the same "ivy paste." The patches were removed in 2-3 days and observed 1 week after application. Of 48, 32 reacted to the challenge test (67%). Strauss retested 6 of the 16 negatives, and 3 of these were reactive on the second challenge. This is how he achieved his final figure of 35 sensitized of 48. However, since the same potent extract was used for challenge and sensitization, 3 of the positive reactors actually underwent 2 sensitization procedures. Spontaneous flareup of sensitization sites was not mentioned.

Can premature neonates be sensitized? Uhr et al. [2] attempted to sensitize premature neonates to dinitrofluorobenzene by applying 0.02-0.04 ml of a 10% solution in acetone. They patch tested with 0.01 M dinitrofluorobenzene in corn oil-acetone. The patch tests were removed and read after 2 days. They tested older infants and full-term neonates in addition to premature neonates weighing an average of 1255 g. All 5 infant controls (age 2-12 months) were sensitized. Of 5 full-term neonates, 2 were sensitized. Of 10 premature neonates, 3 were sensitized. A footnote states that 2 of 3 sensitized premature neonates received a second sensitizing dose 9 days after the first; there is no mention of a second sensitizing procedure elsewhere in their paper.

W. L. Epstein [3] tested the sensitization potential of 102 infants and children between the ages of 1 month and 8 years. For sensitization, he applied 0.25 ml of an acetone solution of pentadecyl catechol (PDC), a purified allergen found in dermatitis producing plants of the genus *Rhus*. The sensitizing concentration of PDC was not specified. However it produced a primary irritant reaction in all subjects.

The subjects were challenged 1 month later with 1% PDC in acetone. The tests were covered with a bandage for 2 days and read 4-6 days after application. Children below 1 year of age (results were tabulated by age in years) were less easily sensitized than older children; their positive reactions were less intense. Of 27 children under 1 year, 12 (44%) were sensitized as opposed to 34 of 39 (87%) of those 3-8 years old. The 1-3 year age group had an intermediate incidence of sensitization, 15 of 26 (58%) being sensitized.

Cellular immunity (T-cell function) in neonates is a subject of intense research and a current review by Stiehm et al. [4]. However, we were unable to find any recent study on experimental contact sensitization in the neonate.

REACTIVITY OF NEONATAL SKIN AND ITS SIGNIFICANCE FOR PATCH TESTING

During the first few months of life, human skin shows a marked decrease in reactivity to foreign materials. This field is of great current research interest, and has been recently reviewed in a symposium on Host Defenses in the Fetus and Neonate [5]. Most of the older research is centered on the cutaneous response to intradermal testing. Earlier studies on the relative skin "anergy" of neonates to intracutaneous tests were briefly reviewed by Tschertkow in 1929 [6].

We are concerned with the response of neonatal and infant skin to contactants and the implications for patch testing in these age groups. Adelsberger in 1927 [7] showed that the irritant response to patch tests with turpentine varied greatly with age during the first year of life. She employed closed 4-hr patch tests with *undiluted* turpentine, reading the results at 24 hr. While only 11% of those aged 0-3 months reacted, 52% of infants aged 6-12 months had positive reactions. Those aged 3-6 months showed 34% positive reactions.

Rockl et al. [8] patch tested 357, mostly healthy, children aged 1 month to 14 years with six materials often causing contact dermatitis in adults. The test

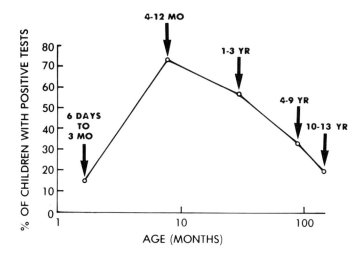

Figure 1 Percentage of children with positive patch tests to one or more test substances at different ages. (*Source*: Ref. 8.)

agents were 0.5% potassium dichromate, 0.1% mercury bichloride, 1.2% formalin, 2% nickel sulfate, 5% turpentine, and 5% benzocaine. The percentage of positive reactions varied with the test substance and age. Potassium dichromate produced the most reaction (29.7%) and benzocaine the fewest (0.8%). The authors interpret the reactions as being irritant responses and noted a striking variation with age. They plotted the number of children reacting to one or more substances against the age; the results are reproduced in Figure 1. While only 15.4% of those aged 3 months or less reacted, 72.8% of those aged 4-12 months had positive tests. After 1 year of age the percentage of positive reactors gradually decreased.

Marcussen [9] patch tested children aged 0-10 years with 5% nickel sulfate and 4% formalin. Twenty-nine percent had positive test reactions to nickel and 20% to formalin. Figure 2 illustrates his data and shows the positive reactives were maximal at age 1 year and diminish progressively to age 8. No reactions were seen in children older than age 8. The age distribution of the infants below 1 year of age was not given.

Marcussen believed these to be irritant and *not* allergic tests. He concluded that patch tests with children require weaker dilutions of allergens than those used for adults. He had tested the children with 1% nickel sulfate and, since none reacted, suggested that 1% nickel sulfate was an appropriate test concentration for children.

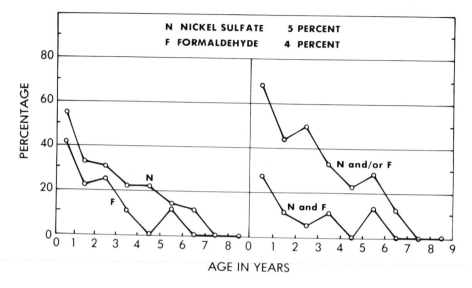

Figure 2 Percentage of primary irritant reactions to nickel sulfate 5% and formaldehyde 4% in children of different age groups. (*Source*: Ref. 9, copyright 1963, American Medical Association.)

Muller and Rockl in 1975 [10] reviewed their earlier work and the findings of others. They concluded that the standard patch test concentrations used for adults are not suitable for testing children since they frequently produce irritant reactions. They pointed out that determining appropriate patch test concentrations for children would be exceedingly difficult in view of the age variation in response to irritants.

CLINICAL SIGNIFICANCE OF ALLERGIC CONTACT DERMATITIS IN NEONATES

The phrase "allergic contact dermatitis" is emphasized since contact dermatitis is sometimes used to describe eruptions produced by contact with irritants. Dermatitis from irritants is common to all age groups and frequent in young infants and small children.

Contact dermatitis in neonates and infants appears to be exceedingly rare, although there are no studies on its prevalence. Muller and Rockl [10] emphasized that some earlier reports on contact allergy in children misinterpreted irritant patch test responses to allergens designed for testing adults.

Contact sensitization depends on two factors: (1) a subject capable of sensitization and (2) appropriate exposure to a potential allergen. In U.S. Adults the common causes of allergic contact dermatitis are: Plants belonging to the rhus family, nickel, topical medicaments, rubber chemicals, perfumes, and chromates. With the exception of topical medicaments, infants are unlikely to come into contact with these substances.

In North America acute contact contact dermatitis from rhus family plants is common in small children, often after they have played outdoors in areas infested with these plants. Nickel allergy affects approximately 10% of adult women in North America and Finland [11,12]. Jewelry and ear-piercing are the apparent sources of sensitization and are hardly a risk for the neonate.

Although allergic contact dermatitis in neonates and small infants is unusual, an occasional case may be overlooked since patch testing is rarely done in this age group. Neonates and small infants can be sensitized. The lack of contact sensitization in this age group is a consequence of the lack of exposure to the more potent allergens in our environment.

Note added in proof: After submission of this paper, Hjorth published an excellent short review on contact dermatitis in children (see Ref. 13).

REFERENCES

1. Straus HW: Artificial sensitization of infants to poison ivy. J Allergy 2: 137-144, 1931.
2. Uhr JW, Dancis J, Neumann CG: Delayed-type hypersensitivity in premature neonatal humans. Nature 187:1130, 1960.
3. Epstein WL: Contact-type delayed hypersensitivity in infants and children: induction of rhus sensitivity. Pediatrics 27:51-53, 1961.
4. Stiehm ER, Winter HS, Bryson YJ: Cellular (T cell) immunity in the human newborn. Pediatrics 64 [Suppl:814-821, 1979.
5. Symposium on host defenses in the fetus and neonate. Pediatrics 64 [Suppl]: 705-833 (November) 1979.
6. Tschertkow L: Ueber die hautanergie bei sauglingen. Z Immun Forsch 64: 407-412, 1929.
7. Adelsberger L: Das verhalten der kindlichen haut gegenuber verschiedenen reizen. Z Kinderheilk 43:373-390, 1927.
8. Rockl H, Muller E, Hilterman W: Zum aussagewert positiver epicutantests bei sauglingen und kindern. Arch Klin Exp Dermatol 226:407-419, 1966.
9. Marcussen, PV: Primary irritant patch-test reactions in children. Arch Dermatol 87:378-382, 1963.
10. Muller E, Rockl H: Aussagewert von lappchentests bei kindern und jugendlichen. Hautarzt 26:85-87, 1975.
11. Prystowsky SD, Allen AM, Smith RW, et al: Allergic contact hypersensitivity to nickel, neomycin, ethylenediamine, and benzocaine. Arch Dermatol 115:959-962, 1979.
12. Peltonen L: Nickel sensitivity in the general population. Contact Dermatitis 5:27-32, 1979.
13. Hjorth N: Contact dermatitis in children. Acta Dermatovener (Stockholm) Suppl. 95:36-39 (1981).

17

Effects of Prolonged Skin Occlusion

RAZA ALY and HOWARD MAIBACH
University of California Medical School, San Francisco, California

Diaper dermatitis (diaper rash) has captivated the curiosity of numerous investigators (see Chap. 14). Although many specific entities (e.g., candidiasis) have been lumped together under this description, it is likely that one critical factor in its pathogenesis relates to occlusion or semi-occlusion: "primitive" societies not utilizing diapers have fewer problems in this regard.

Model systems in humans and animal are needed to aid identification and explanation of the effects of occlusion on skin. Our 5 day human skin occlusion method is one approach to this question.

The ability of skin to control its colonization of bacteria may be due to factors such as bacterial antagonism [1,2] skin lipids and dessication [3-7]. Many pathogenic microorganisms such as hemolytic streptococci and *Staphylococcus aureus*, when artificially applied, do not survive for more than a few hours. Yet, on some, these organisms survive, multiply, and even produce disease. The normal flora is denser in moist intertriginous regions [8]. Most of the water on the skin is derived from eccrine sweat and transepidermal water loss. In the axillary region there is also intermittent contribution from apocrine sweat.

Marples demonstrated the effect of hydration on the bacterial flora of the skin using several occlusive devices [9]. All methods greatly increased the number of organisms. Other factors such as transepidermal water loss (TEWL), pH, and CO_2 emission rates were not quantitatively measured. We measured the effect of complete occlusion of the skin on various parameters such as the aerobic microbial flora, pH, transepidermal water loss, and CO_2 emission rate.

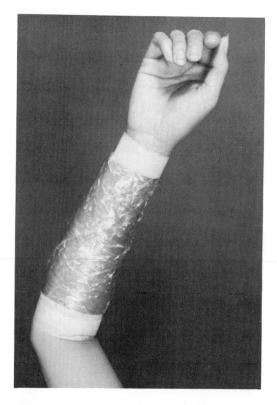

Figure 1   The arm was occluded with a plastic film (Saran Wrap) for 5 days. This film was tightly secured at the wrist and just below the elbow with paper adhesive tape (Micropore).

BACTERIA UNDER OCCLUSION

Ten healthy male and female volunteers, working in similar laboratory environments, were included. They did not use germicidal soap for 7 days before and during the investigation.

Their arms were wrapped with plastic film Saran Wrap for 5 days (Fig. 1). Each day a succeeding portion of the wrap was removed to take measurements and microbial samples. Bacterial samples were removed by the detergent scrub method [10] and identified by appropriate biochemical methods [11,12].

The total average geometric microbial counts before occlusion were 1.8×10^2 organisms/cm^2; this increased dramatically after 24 hr of occlusion to 1.4×10^6/cm (Fig. 2). Maximum counts (9.8×10^7/cm^2) were noted on day 4 of occlusion.

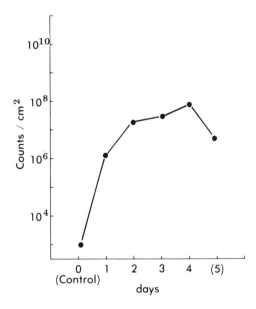

Figure 2 Total geometric microbial counts/cm^2 under occlusion. The skin was occluded for 5 days. The counts before occlusion were considered as control. (*Source*: from Ref. 6. © 1978, The Williams & Wilkins Co., Baltimore.)

The types of microorganisms comprising the total counts changed (Fig. 3). The coagulase-negative staphylococci counts peaked on day 4. The maximum counts for micrococci on day 3 were 9.9×10^4/cm^2; this reduced dramatically on days 4 and 5 in spite of continued occlusion. Lipophilic coryneforms were not detected before occlusion; they peaked on day 5 (1.5×10^5/cm^2), remaining the second highest flora on days 4 and 5. Lipophilic coryneform prefer a higher pH and moister environment than micrococci. There were no definite trends for coryneforms because they fluctuated day-to-day.

Gram-negative rods emerged after occlusion but never became the dominant flora. In Marples' study [9], gram-negative rods increased to 10% of the total flora after 4 days of occlusion. In our study, gram-negatives were less than 1% of the total flora. Neither coagulase-positive staphylococci nor B hemolytic streptococci appeared after occlusion. No occluded areas demonstrated *Pseudomonas aeruginosa*.

SKIN PH UNDER OCCLUSION

The skin pH remains fairly constant in the normal adult population; most skin bacteria can grow under all pH conditions found on the skin. A slight change in

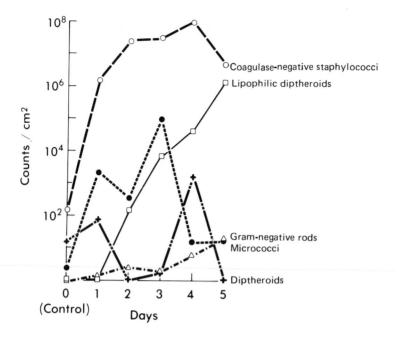

Figure 3 Geometric microbial counts/cm^2 under the occlusion. The counts before occlusion were considered as control. (*Source*: from Ref. 6. © 1978, The Williams & Wilkins Co., Baltimore.)

pH might cause an ecological advantage in growth rate for a particular organism with regard to its optimum hydrogen ion concentration. A pH meter (Beckman Electromate) was used to measure the skin's pH before and after occlusion (Fig. 4). The pH of the skin gradually shifted from the acidic range (4.38) before occlusion, to neutral (7.05) on day 4 of occlusion. The pH of the skin may have reached an equilibrium with the interstitial fluid, as the final pH was close to the body pH. In general, skin pH is higher in humid intertriginous areas.

TRANSEPIDERMAL WATER LOSS UNDER OCCLUSION

Transepidermal water loss (TEWL) was measured with an electrolytic water analyzer (Fig. 4). TEWL reflects water diffusing through the moist membranes of the analyzer and water being lost as part of hydration. Increased TEWL reflects increase in water content of skin surface provided no damage has occurred. TEWL was 0.56 mg/cm^2/hr before occlusion and increased to 1.87 mg/cm^2/hr

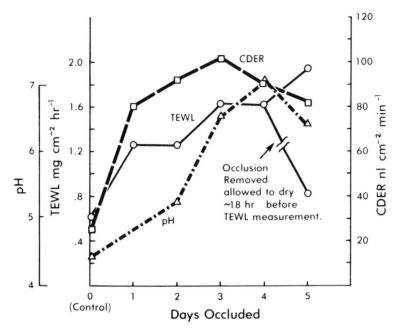

Figure 4 Effect of occlusion on transepidermal water loss (TEWL), carbon dioxide emission rate (CDER), and pH of skin. The unoccluded skin served as control. (*Source*: from Ref. 6. © 1978, The Williams & Wilkins Co., Baltimore.)

on day 5. With occlusion the skin was essentially saturated within 24 hr. TEWL was measured 18 hr after removal of occlusion to determine if there was any structural damage to the skin. These values, although higher than for previously occluded skin, were not significantly different from the control.

CARBON DIOXIDE EMISSION RATE UNDER OCCLUSION

The carbon dioxide emission rate (CDER), measured with an infrared analyzer, increased from less than 0.1% to more than 5% (Fig. 4). Changes in concentrations have effects on the type of microbial flora if two types are grown in competition [13].

Normally, CO_2 passes through the skin and into the atmosphere with little chance of building up local concentrations. Previous investigations have shown that, after a few hours, the CO_2 concentration under occlusion (such as Saran Wrap) approaches equilibrium with underlying tissues. The resulting atmosphere contains about 5-7% CO_2.

In summary, skin occlusion with plastic film influences several skin factors. Some of these were measured in this investigation. Other factors such as nutrients, bacterial metabolites, bacterial antagonisms, skin surface lipids, and salt concentration may have been changed with this occlusion, exerting an accumulative pressure on the skin biota. These data are complex and not easily interpreted. This is the longest-term occlusion data presently available in which a broad attempt was made to profile the physiological changes involved.

This data was obtained on adults; similar studies should be done in infants from birth to several months of age. Following the flora serially (qualitatively and quantitatively) and related factors described here should provide additional leads and insights into the pathogenesis of diaper dermatitis.

This study, the most complex of its type yet undertaken, provides some insight into the complexity of the effects of occlusion on skin. We must certainly investigate the mechanisms controlling the dramatic appearance of lipophilic coryneforms and the less dramatic but equally important arrival of gram-negatives.

We must also investigate other physiologic and biochemical changes produced by occlusion if we are to improve our understanding (and prophylaxis) of diaper dermatitis.

REFERENCES

1. Marsh PD, Selwyn S: Studies on antagonism between human skin bacteria. J Med Microbiol 10:161-169, 1977.
2. Selwyn S: Natural antibiosis among skin bacteria as a primary defense against infection. Br J Dermatol 93:487-493, 1975.
3. Aly R, Maibach H, Shinefield H, Strauss W: Survival of pathogenic microorganisms on human skin. J Invest Dermatol 58:205-210, 1972.
4. Burtenshaw JM: The autogenous disinfection of skin, in *Modern Trend in Dermatology,* edited by R. M. B. Mackenna. Butterworth and Co., Ltd., London, 1948.
5. Aly R, Maibach H, Rahman R, Shinefield H, Mandel A: Correlation of human in vivo and in vitro cutaneous antimicrobial factors. J Infect Dis 131:579-583, 1975.
6. Aly R, Shirley C, Cunico B, Maibach H: Effect of prolonged occlusion on the microbial flora, pH, CO_2 and transepidermal water loss on human skin. J Invest Dermatol 71:378-381, 1978.
7. Rebell G, Pillsbury DM, Phalle G, deSaint M, Ginsberg D: Factors affecting the rapid disappearance of bacteria placed on the normal skin. J Invest Dermatol 14:247-263, 1950.
8. Aly R, Maibach HI: Aerobic microbial flora of intertrigenous skin. Appl Environ Microbiol 33:97-100, 1977.
9. Marples RR: The effect of hydration on the bacterial flora of the skin, in

Skin Bacteria and Their Role in Infection, edited by HI Maibach and Hildic-Smith McGraw-Hill, New York, 1965, pp 33-41.

10. Williamson P, Kligman AM: A new method for quantitative investigation of cutaneous bacteria. J Invest Dermatol 45:498-503, 1965.

11. Stokes EJ: Identification of bacteria, in *Clinical Bacteriology.* Edward, Arnold, London, 1968, pp 89-139.

12. Evans JB, Kloos WE: Use of shake cultures in a semisolid thioglycolate medium for differentiating staphylococci from micrococci. Appl Microbiol 23:326-331, 1972.

13. King RD, Dillavou CL, Greenberg JH, Jeppsen JC, and Jaeger JS: Identification of CO_2 as a dermatophyte inhibitory factory produced by *C. albicans.* Can J Microbiol 22:1720-1727, 1976.

CLINICAL ASPECTS

18

Cutaneous Diseases of the Newborn

SIDNEY HURWITZ

Yale University School of Medicine, New Haven, Connecticut

The skin of the infant differs from that of the adult in that it is thinner, less hairy, has weaker intercellular attachments, and produces fewer sweat and sebaceous gland secretions. Although much has been published on the various disorders and phenomena peculiar to the integument of infants, it is unfortunate that very little is known about the physiologic variations and reactivity of the skin in neonates. As a result, the skin of the neonate presents a broad area for future research and investigation [1,2].

Diseases of the skin in newborns often presents patterns which diverge from those of the same disease in adults (Table 1). There are certain increased vulnerabilities to bacterial, viral, and physiochemical insults, and a few cutaneous diseases peculiar to children. Some of the anatomic and physiologic reasons for these differences are apparent, but others are entirely unknown or can only be conjectured [3].

Inflammatory contact dermatitis in infants is more likely to be due to primary irritant effect than to sensitization. True eczematous sensitivity to external contactants is rarely present in the newborn. The infant apparently has not yet been stimulated to the formation of specific antibodies for the production of atopic reactions. Infants below the age of 1 year have a markedly depressed ability to react to allergens, children between 1 and 3 have an intermediate ability, and children between 3 and 8 years are readily sensitized and show a depth of sensitivity and intensity of reaction comparable to that seen in adults [4,5]. The decreased reactivity of infant skin to certain allergens, although not completely

Table 1 Characteristics of Neonatal Skin Compared With
Adult Skin

1. Thinner, less hairy, weaker intercellular attachments
2. Fewer eccrine and sebaceous gland secretions
3. Increased susceptibility to external irritants
4. Increased susceptibility to micrococcal infection
5. Depressed contact allergen reactivity
6. Percutaneous permeability increased only in premature babies, damaged or scrotal skin

Source: Ref. 2.

understood, appears to be related to a decreased function of cellular-mediated immune mechanism and the decreased exposure of infants and young children to potential sensitizing allergens.

It has been theorized that newborn skin is more susceptible to external irritants. This remains controversial and requires further investigation. Irritating chemical substances such as detergents, talc, excessive washing, chafing, and prolonged exposure to cold and wind are more common causes of eczematous eruption than allergy to food or topically applied agents. In irritant dermatitis the site of eruption varies with the etiologic agents. Saliva may be irritating to the face and chin, fecal secretions irritate the buttocks, and topical preparations in adequate concentration may cause a dermatitis in infants but may not necessarily affect older individuals when used in the same concentrations.

For years physicians have considered newborn skin to be more susceptible to the percutaneous absorption of potential toxic substances. Current data, however, reveal that although the skin of the premature infant is indeed more permeable, undamaged skin of normal full-term newborns (except for the scrotal area) is no more susceptible to percutaneous absorption than that of older children or adults [6]. The problem of percutaneous permeability and absorption in infancy, therefore, is one of greater relative ratio of skin surface to body volume in infants and small children (as compared to that of older children and adults). This, accordingly, results in the risk of higher blood level accumulation of potential toxic substances in this age group.

The skin acts as a protective organ. Any break in its integrity affords an opportunity for initiation of infection. Skin care of the newborn is complicated by the fact that the infant does not have the protective skin flora at birth, has at least one and possibly two open surgical wounds (the umbilicus and circumcision sites), and is exposed to fomites and personnel that may harbor a variety of infectious agents [7]. A discussion of the inflammatory response in newborns,

Table 2 Host Defenses in Human Neonates

1. Impaired movement and bactericidal activity of neutrophils and monocytes
2. Decreased opsonization with lower C_3 and C_5 levels
3. Increased susceptibility to monilial, micrococcal, and viral infection

Source: Data from Ref. 8.

as in adults, can be divided into two aspects: cellular and humoral. Cellular aspects include polymorphonuclear leukocytes and monocytes; humoral aspects include the opsonins, serum bactericidal substances, and chemotactic factors. The neutrophils and monocytes of the newborn differ from those of the adult in many ways. Cell movement is severely impaired in the newborn. In addition, the bactericidal activity of neutrophils is deficient in the newborn suggesting that they may have "burned themselves out" during the birth process. Humoral aspects of the inflammatory response are also greatly deficient in the newborn with a deficit in opsonization. The major deficiency seems to be in the complement system: serum levels of C_3 and C_5 are low and therefore the opsonins generated from activation of these two complement components are low. The presence of this combination of deficiencies is more than adequate to explain the increased susceptibility of newborns to infectious diseases (Table 2) [8,9].

TOXIC ERYTHEMA NEONATORUM

Toxic erythema of the newborn represents a characteristic, asymptomatic, benign, self-limited cutaneous eruption during the neonatal period of unknown etiology. Erythematous macules, papules, pustules, or a combination of these lesions may occur anywhere on the body (except the palms and soles) and may vary in number from a few (two or three) to several hundred. That these lesions are not seen on the palms and soles is explained by the absence of pilosebaceous follicles in these regions (Table 3).

The eruption may first appear as a blotchy macular erythema which may develop into firm, 1-3 mm, pale yellow or white papules, pustules, or a combination of these lesions on an erythematous base; the so-called "flea-bitten" rash of the newborn (Fig. 1). The erythematous macules generally display an irregular or splotchy appearance varying in size from a few millimeters to several centimeters in diameter. They may be seen in sharp contrast to the surrounding unaffected skin, may blend into a surrounding erythema, or progress to a confluent eruption.

Although erythema toxicum appears most frequently during the first 3-4 days of life, it may be seen at birth, or as late as the 10th day of life. Exacerbations and remissions may occur during the first 2 weeks of life. The duration of indi-

Table 3 Toxic Erythema Neonatorum

1. Incidence: 30-70% of infants (increases with maturity)
2. Multiple 1-3 mm pale yellow or white papules, pustules, or combinations, on an erythematous base
3. Spares palms and soles
4. Diagnosis
    Eosinophils on Wright's or Giemsa stain
    Biopsy: eosinophils about pilosebaceous structures
5. Etiology? (an eosinophilic response to trauma?)

Source: Data from Ref. 2.

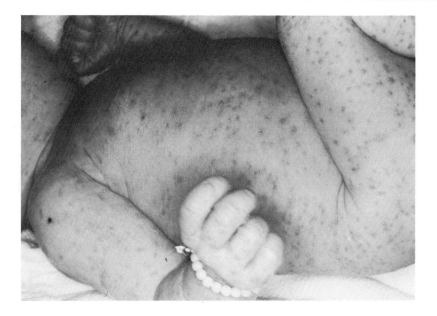

Figure 1 Toxic erythema of the newborn (erythema toxicum neonatorum). A combination of blotchy macular erythema and 1 to 3 mm pale yellow or white papules and pustules on an erythematous base: the so-called "flea-bitten" rash of the newborn. (*Source*: Ref. 2.)

vidual lesions may vary from a few hours to 16 days (the average duration is approximately 2 days).

Its reported incidence is variable due to the fleeting nature of the disorder and the disparity of the lesions and clinical observations on the part of clinicians. Some authors report an incidence as low as 4.5%, others report incidences varying from 31 to 70% of newborns. The incidence does not differ significantly with respect to maternal history, condition at birth, or sex. It does, however, have a lower rate of incidence in premature as contrasted to full-term infants, with an increase in incidence (from 0 to 59%) as the gestational age increases (from 30 weeks or less to 42 weeks or more) [10]. Studies of the acute inflammatory process in newborns reveal an eosinophilic response suggesting that eosinophilia may be a normal newborn response to the stimulus of injury [11]. At present the etiology of erythema toxicum remains obscure. It may represent a transient reaction of newborn skin to normal mechanical or thermal stimuli [11].

TRANSIENT NEONATAL PUSTULAR MELANOSIS

Transient neonatal pustular melanosis is a recently recognized vesiculopustular and pigmented disorder of newborns first described in 1976 (Table 4). Seen in 4.4% of black and 0.2% of white newborns it is characterized by superficial vesiculopustular lesions which rupture easily and evolve into evanescent pinhead-sized hyperpigmented macules [12].

These lesions are usually present at birth. They generally begin as superficial vesiculopustular lesions which rupture easily during the first bathing and often leave a collarette of fine white scales that surround a pinhead-sized brown hyperpigmented macule which generally fades within a period of several weeks to months. The lesions most often are seen in clusters under the chin, on the forehead, nape of the neck, lower back, and shins. Occasionally, lesions also may

Table 4 Transient Neonatal Pustular Melanosis

1. 4.4% of black, 0.2% of white newborns
2. Superficial vesiculopustules
   Forehead, nape of neck, lower back, shins
   (occasionally cheeks and trunk)
   Histology: Intracorneal and subcorneal pustules
3. Hyperpigmented macules
   Basketweave hyperkeratosis
   Histology: Focal basilar hyperpigmentation

Source: Data from Ref. 12.

appear on the cheeks, trunk, and extremities. Rarely, blisters, which do not progress to pigmented macules, may be detected on the scalp, palms, and soles.

Transient neonatal pustular melanosis is a benign disorder, appears to have no associated systemic manifestations, and requires no treatment. Lesions appear to be different from those of erythema toxicum and must be differentiated from those pustulovesicles of staphylococcal or herpetic origin. Vesiculopustular lesions of transient neonatal pustular melanosis disappear in 24-28 hr, often leaving hyperpigmented pinhead-size macules which in turn generally regress within 3 weeks to 3 months.

HERPES SIMPLEX NEONATORUM

The skin and mucous membranes of the infant are sometimes peculiarly susceptible to primary infection to the herpes simplex virus, with the production of an intense local reaction and serious systemic symptoms. Disseminated herpes virus hominis simplex infection in the newborn generally is thought to be associated with grave prognosis for mortality and severe neurological sequelae among survivors. Current evidence, however, reveals that herpes simplex infection in young infants may result in a broad spectrum of illness ranging from death or recovery with severe central nervous system or ocular damage to mild or asymptomatic infection with apparent complete recovery [13]. Neonatal herpetic infection may be categorized as disseminated, local, or asymptomatic. The relative frequency of the various forms of neonatal infection is unknown. More than half the newborns with herpes simplex infection have skin manifestations and about one-half of infected infants, if untreated, will die or suffer serious neurological or ocular sequelae.

The clinical picture of herpes simplex neonatorum frequently is that of a previously apparently well baby who becomes ill on the 4th to 8th day of life, when vesicular lesions may be detected on the skin or buccal mucosa. The eruption may vary from erythematous, flat, or depressed lesions to individual grouped vesicles or a widespread generalized vesicobullous eruption on the skin or buccal mucosa (Fig. 2). Skin lesions occur most often on the scalp and face, the areas closest to and in longest contact with the cervical area from which the infection is transmitted during normal childbirth. When cutaneous lesions are absent, disseminated neonatal herpes infection may be confused with sepsis, toxoplasmosis, or cytomegalic inclusion disease. The diagnosis of herpesvirus infection of the newborn accordingly may be aided by Tzanck test, viral culture, or biopsy of cutaneous lesions.

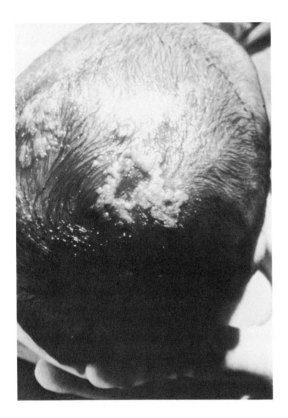

Figure 2 Individual grouped vesicles on the scalp of a newborn infant with herpes simplex neonatorum. (*Source*: Ref. 2.)

IMPETIGO NEONATORUM

The great susceptibility of newborn skin to micrococcal infection was graphically demonstrated in epidemics in nurseries before the availability of adequate bacterial drugs. These widespread superficial infections, unfortunately all too frequently fatal, were variously called impetigo, "pemphigus neonatorum," or Ritter's disease.

Impetigo in newborns may occur as early as the 2nd or 3rd day, or as late as the 2nd week of life. It usually presents as a superficial vesicular, pustular, or

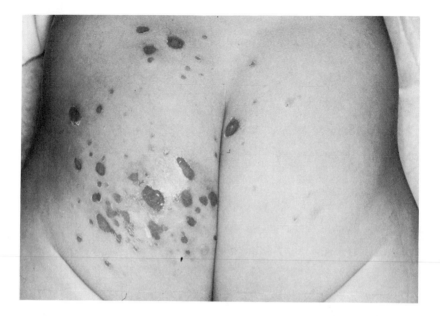

Figure 3 Denuded bullae on an erythematous base associated with a staphylococcal pyroderma.

bullous lesion on an erythematous base (Fig. 3). Vesicles are easily denuded leaving a round, red, raw moist surface, usually without crust formation. Blisters often are wrinkled, contain some fluid, and are easily denuded without formation of crusts. "Pemphigus neonatorum" is an archaic misnomer occasionally applied to superficial bullous lesions of severe impetigo widely distributed over the surface of the body. The status of "pemphigus neonatorum" as a distinct nosologic entity is dubious. Fortunately, with improved neonatal care and appropriate antibiotic therapy, this severe form of neonatal pyoderma rarely is seen today.

TOXIC EPIDERMAL NECROLYSIS

Toxic epidermal necrolysis (TEN) is a specific exfoliative dermatitis consisting of two separate and distinct entities. The overwhelming majority of cases in infants and children are caused by an exfoliative toxin ("exfoliatin") generally caused by coagulase-positive group II staphylococci, usually but not necessarily phage type 55 or 71. This form is often termed staphylococcal scalded skin syndrome (SSSS) [14]. The reason for the increased incidence in infants and young children appears to be related to the fact that adults and 85% of children

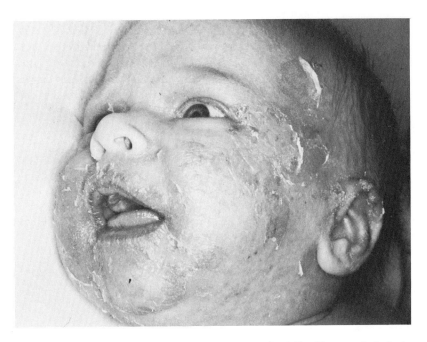

Figure 4 Staphylococcal scalded skin syndrome (SSSS). Characteristic facies with crusting, perioral fissures, and erythema. Note peeling of the epidermis on the forehead and cheek caused by pressure (Nikolsky's sign). (*Source*: Ref. 2.)

over 10 years of age have specific antistaphylococcal antibody which allows the development of localized staphylococcal bullous impetigo but limits blood stream dissemination of toxin in older persons.

In older children and adults, toxic epidermal necrolysis is usually, but not necessarily, related to a hypersensitivity to drugs. The reason for the decreased incidence of drug-induced toxic epidermal necrolysis in infants and young children remains unknown.

Staphylococcal scalded skin syndrome often begins with a prodromal period of malaise, fever, and irritability; a generalized erythema with a fine, stippled sandpaper appearance; and exquisite tenderness of the skin. From the intertriginous and periorificial areas, and trunk, the erythema and tenderness spread over the entire body, but usually spare the hairy parts. Children are extremely irritable, uncomfortable, and difficult to hold, due to the extreme tenderness of the skin. Within 2 or 3 days, frequently in a few hours, the upper layer of epidermis may become wrinkled or may be removed (often peeling off like wet tissue paper) by light stroking, the characteristic Nikolsky's sign (Fig. 4). The patient develops a highly characteristic pathognomonic facies: crusting and perioral erythema with fissures and rhagades about the nasolabial folds and corners of the mouth. Although an occasional patient may be seriously ill, when treated properly most have surprisingly little difficulty except for extreme irritability and skin tenderness. The mortality rate, if untreated, is highest in children under 1 year of age and relatively low in those of 1-6 years of age. Death, when it occurs, usualy has been the result of sepsis and fluid and electrolyte imbalance.

NEONATAL SYPHILIS

The cohesion of the dermo-epidermal junction in infants is apparently less firm than in adults, and certain diseases which rarely or never produce bullous reactions in the adult may do so in the child. Impetigo tends to be bullous in infants and children and congenital syphilis seen in the newborn may induce bullous lesions of the skin, which almost never occurs in the adult.

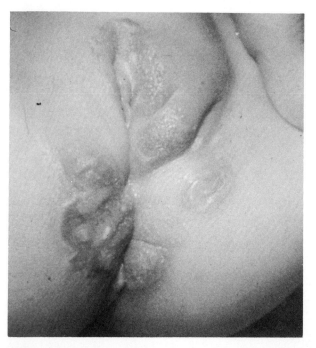

Figure 5 Congenital syphilis. Eroded lesions in the genital area of an infant with neonatal syphilis. (*Source*: Courtesy of Dr. Gabriela Lowy, Rio de Janiero, Brazil.)

As a result of advances in the detection and treatment of syphilis during the years following the Second World War, the incidence of neonatal syphilis dropped to relatively insignificant levels by the mid-1950s. Since 1959, however, the incidence of primary and secondary syphilis has increased with a resultant resurgence in the incidence of congenital syphilis (a disorder which to a generation of physicians had been well-documented but temporarily forgotten) [15]. During the past 2 years, however, it is gratifying to note that, despite the increased incidence of primary syphilis in women, congenital syphilis again is in decline, probably as the result of increased surveillance of pregnant women.

Fetal infection with *Treponema pallidum* results in multiple system involvement with considerable variation in the clinical expression. Although infants with congenital syphilis may exhibit no external evidence of disease at birth, the majority show clinical manifestations in the 1st month of life.

Cutaneous lesions of congenital syphilis may be seen in one-third to one-half of affected infants. They may be quite varied in character, but most commonly appear as large round or oval maculopapular or papulosquamous lesions comparable to those seen in secondary syphilis of the adolescent or adult (Fig. 5). The

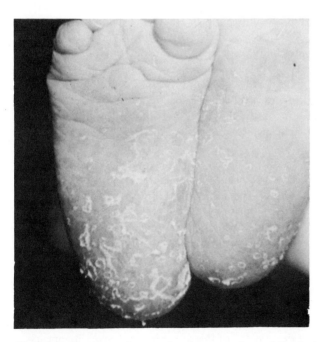

Figure 6 Desquamation on the plantar surface of the feet of an infant with neonatal syphilis. (*Source*: Courtesy of Dr. Gabriela Lowy, Rio de Janiero, Brazil.)

eruption may appear on any part of the body, usually is most pronounced on the face, dorsal surface of the trunk and legs, diaper area, and, at times, the palms and soles. Vesiculobullous hemorrhagic lesions of congenital syphilis occasionally are present at birth but more frequently develop in the first few days of life and, especially when seen on the palms and soles, are highly diagnostic of this disorder (Fig. 6). Blisters appear on an area of dusky redness, are of irregular size, and contain a cloudy or hemorrhagic liquid teeming with spirochetes [1]. The palms and soles may be fissured, erythematous, and, due to subcutaneous edema, indurated with a dull red, shiny, almost polished appearance. Concomitant with these changes is desquamation of the skin in large flakes over the entire body. Even when not present elsewhere, this desquamation still may be detected around the nails of the fingers and toes of affected infants.

SCLEREMA NEONATORUM AND SUBCUTANEOUS FAT NECROSIS

Skin turgor at birth generally is normal during the first few hours of life. As normal physiologic dehydration occurs (up to 10% of birth weight) during the first 3 or 4 days of life, the skin generally becomes loose and wrinkled in appearance. Subcutaneous fat, normally quite adequate at birth, increases in amount until about 9 months of age, thus accounting for the traditional chubby appearance of the healthy neonate. A decrease or absence of this normal panniculus is abnormal and suggests the possibility of prematurity, postmaturity, or placental insufficiency.

Sclerma neonatorum and subcutaneous fat necrosis appear to be clinical variants of the same disorder or closely allied abnormalities of subcutaneous tissue (Table 5). Although there is considerable confusion in the literature, recent evidence suggests that the biochemical abnormality of these two disorders may be identical.

Sclerema neonatorum is a diffuse, rapidly spreading, waxlike hardening of the skin and subcutaneous tissue which occurs in premature or debilitated infants during the first few weeks of life. The disorder, usually associated with a serious underlying condition such as sepsis or other infection, congenital heart disease, respiratory distress, diarrhea, or dehydration, is characterized by a diffuse nonpitting woody induration of the involved tissues. The process is symmetrical, usually starting on the legs and buttocks, and may progress to involve all areas except the palms, soles, and genitalia. As the disorder spreads the skin becomes cold, yellowish-white, mottled, stony hard, and cadaverlike. The limbs become immobile and the face acquires a fixed masklike expression. The infants become sluggish, feed poorly, show clinical signs of shock, and, in a high percentage of cases often die. Although the etiology of this disorder is unknown, it appears to represent a nonspecific sign of grave prognostic significance rather than a pri-

Table 5 Characteristic Differences Between Sclerema Neonatorum and Subcutaneous Fat Necrosis

Sclerema neonatorum	Subcutaneous fat necrosis
1. Serious underlying disease (sepsis, coronary heart disease, respiratory distress, diarrhea, or dehydration)	1. Healthy newborns
2. Waxlike hardening of skin and subcutaneous tissue in premature or debilitated infants	2. Circumscribed indurated and nodular areas of fat necrosis
3. Etiology: hypothermia, peripheral chilling with vascular collapse, defect in fatty acid mobilization?	3. Etiology: pressure on bony prominences during delivery, asphyxia, hypothermia, or maternal diabetes
4. Histology: edema and thickening of CT bands around fat lobules, needle-shaped clefts within fat cells	4. Histology: large fat lobules, inflammatory infiltrate in subcutaneous tissue, foreign body giant cells around crystals of fatty acid
5. Management: supportive care, heat, O_2, control of infection, iv fluids, systemic steroids	5. Management: most resolve spontaneously in 2–4 weeks; aspiration of fluctuant lesions as required.

Source: Ref. 2.

mary disease [16]. Exposure to cold, hypothermia, peripheral chilling with vascular collapse, and an increase in the ratio of saturated to unsaturated fatty acids in the triglyceride fraction of the subcutaneous tissue (due to a defect in fatty acid mobilization) have been suggested but lack confirmation as possible causes for this disorder [17].

The prognosis of sclerema neonatorum is generally poor and mortality occurs in 50-75% of affected infants. Death, when it occurs, generally is due to inanition, debilitation, and the associated underlying pathological disorder. In infants that survive the cutaneous findings resolve without residual sequelae. There is no specific therapy for sclerema neonatorum. Supportive care with heat, oxygen, control of infection, management of the underlying disorder, and intravenous therapy for correction of fluid and electrolyte imbalance is essential. Although indications for their use are unclear and controlled studies fail to confirm their efficacy, in view of the fact that these infants are critically ill and the mortality rate continues to be high, systemic corticosteroids in addition to antimicrobial agents frequently have been advocated.

Subcutaneous fat necrosis is a benign self-limited disease which affects apparently healthy full-term newborns and young infants. It is characterized by

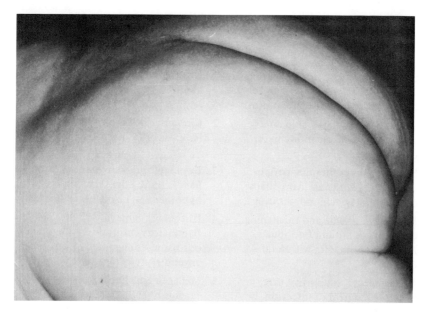

Figure 7 Subcutaneous fat necrosis. Sharply circumscribed reddish to violaceous nodular lesions on the buttocks of an 8-week-old infant.

sharply circumscribed indurated and nodular areas of fat necrosis (Fig. 7). The etiology of this disorder remains unknown but appears to be related to trauma due to pressure on bony prominences during the time of delivery, asphyxia, hypothermia, and, in some instances, maternal diabetes mellitus [18].

The onset of subcutaneous fat necrosis generally occurs in the first few days and weeks of life. Lesions appear as single or multiple localized, sharply circumscribed, usually painless areas of induration. At times, however, infected areas may be extremely tender and infants may be quite uncomfortable and cry vigorously when handled. Lesions of subcutaneous fat necrosis vary in size from small nodules to large plaques and often reach several centimeters in diameter. Although lesions may occur in any cutaneous area, sites of predilection include the cheeks, back, buttocks, arms, and thighs. The involved tissues have a reddish or violaceous hue and a nontender, nonpitting stony consistency. Many lesions have an uneven lobulated surface with an elevated margin separating it from the surrounding normal tissue.

Lesions of subcutaneous fat necrosis tend to have a good prognosis. Although they may develop extensive deposits of calcium which may liquify, drain, and heal with scarring, most areas undergo spontaneous resolution within several weeks. Although many authors consider necrosis and crystallization of the subcutaneous fat to be part of the histopathology of sclerema neonatorum, needle-shaped clefts within cells with necrosis and crystallization of the subcutaneous fat are more characteristic of subcutaneous fat necrosis than sclerema of the newborn.

Most uncomplicated lesions of subcutaneous fat necrosis are self-limited, resolve spontaneously within 2-4 weeks (usually without atrophy or scarring), and accordingly require no specific therapy. Fluctuant lesions, however, should be aspirated with a small-gauge needle to prevent rupture, thus diminishing the possibility of susceptibility to subsequent scarring. Rarely, infants with associated hypercalcemia may require low calcium intake, restriction of vitamin D, and systemic corticosteroid therapy.

ECCRINE AND PILOSEBACEOUS DISORDERS

Differentiation of the epidermis and its appendages, particularly in the premature infant, is frequently incomplete at birth. As a result of this immaturity, a high incidence of sweat-retention phenomena may be seen in the newborn infant. Miliaria, a common neonatal dermatosis caused by sweat retention, is character-

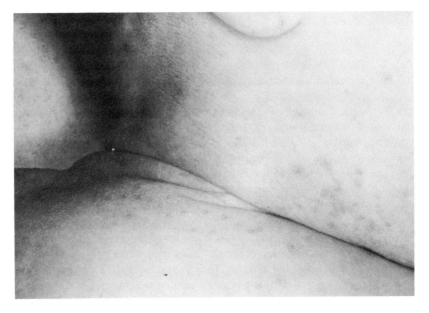

Figure 8   Miliaria rubra on the neck of a 14-day-old infant.

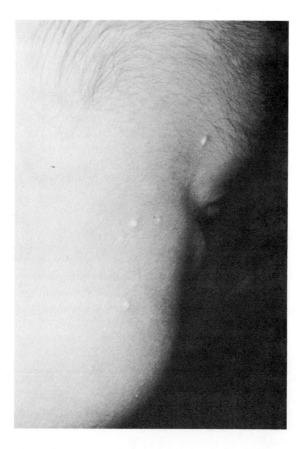

Figure 9 Neonatal milia. Pearly white to yellow papules (1-2 mm) on the face of a 1-month-old infant. (*Source*: Ref. 2.)

ized by a vesicular eruption with subsequent maceration and obstruction of the eccrine ducts (Fig. 8). The pathophysiologic events that lead to this disorder are ketatinous plugging of eccrine ducts and the escape of eccrine sweat into the skin below the level of obstruction.

Milia commonly occur on the face of the newborn. Seen in 40-50% of infants, these result from retention of keratin and sebaceous material within the pilosebaceous apparatus of the neonate. They appear as tiny 1-2 mm pearly white or yellow papules (Fig. 9). Particularly prominent on the cheeks, nose, chin, and forehead, they may be few or numerous and frequently are grouped in the areas of involvement. Although milia of the newborn may persist into the 2nd or 3rd

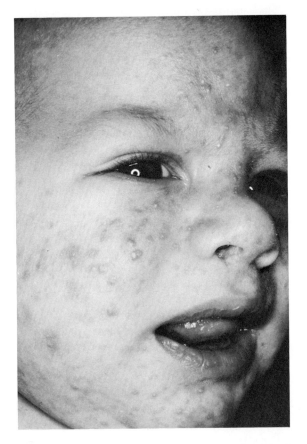

Figure 10 Infantile acne (acne neonatorum) on the face of a 7-week-old infant.

month, they usually disappear spontaneously during the first 3 or 4 weeks of life and, accordingly, require no therapy.

Occasionally, infants develop an eruption which resembles acne vulgaris as seen in adolescents. Although the etiology of acne neonatorum is not clearly defined, it appears to develop as a result of hormonal stimulation of sebaceous glands that have not yet involuted to their childhood state of immaturity. Although testosterone synthesis occurs in the fetal testis and adrenal gland between the 9th and 15th week of intrauterine life, steroid synthesis in the fetal ovary is relatively limited. This may explain the apparent higher incidence of acne neonatorum in male infants [19].

Lesions of acne neonatorum may be present at birth or at any time during the first 3 years of life. They characteristically present as erythematous come-dones, papules, or, occasionally, pustules (Fig. 10). In severe cases cystic and deep-seated nodules have been noted. Lesions are usually confined to the cheeks; occasionally the chin and forehead also may be involved. In contrast to adolescent acne, the chest and back are not affected.

The course of infantile acne may vary considerably. The lesions may be limited to a few comedones which clear after a few weeks. Most cases disappear within the 1st year of life; others reportedly have persisted up to 11 years.

SEBORRHEIC DERMATITIS

Seborrheic dermatitis has been used to describe a self-limiting condition of the scalp, face, ears, trunk, and intertriginous areas characterized by greasy scaling associated with patchy redness, fissuring, and occasional weeping.

The cause of seborrheic dermatitis is not well understood, It appears to be an inflammatory disorder related to dysfunction of the sebaceous glands and has a predilection for areas with a high density of sebaceous glands. Ostensibly under hormonal influence, this disorder first appears during the first few months of infancy when transplacental hormone levels are elevated. It frequently improves between 8 and 12 months of age as these levels decline, only to reappear due to elevation of hormone levels during adolescence. Whether seborrheic dermatitis of adolescence and adulthood is related to that of infancy, however, remains unknown.

LEINER'S DISEASE

Leiner's disease is a rare disorder of infancy characterized by generalized sebor-rheic dermatitis; intractable, severe diarrhea; marked wasting and dystrophy; and recurrent local and systemic infections, usually of gram-negative etiology (Table 6). Many authors now consider this disorder to be an extensive form of sebor-rheic dermatitis of unknown etiology which was described primarily before anti-biotics were available. This disorder may occur during the first week of life, but generally begins suddenly in infants between 2 and 4 months of age. Girls are affected more frequently than boys and the proportion of breast-fed babies is said to be high.

The dermatosis is described as one of universal erythema and loosening of the epidermis with scale and crust formation. Generally considered to be a severe exfoliative variant of seborrheic dermatitis, it commonly begins as a progressive increase in severity of seborrheic dermatitis of the scalp or flexures, or by the sudden development of intense erythema of the entire skin surface with profuse desquamation of fine, branny, scales on the face, heavy crusting of the scalp and

Table 6 Leiner's Disease

1. Onset at age 2-4 months
2. Severe exfoliant seborrheic dermatitis
3. Intractable diarrhea, wasting, and dystrophy
4. Recurrent local and systemic gram-negative infection
5. C_5 dysfunction with decreased opsonic activity
6. Antibiotics, fresh plasma, or whole blood

Source: Data from Ref. 2.

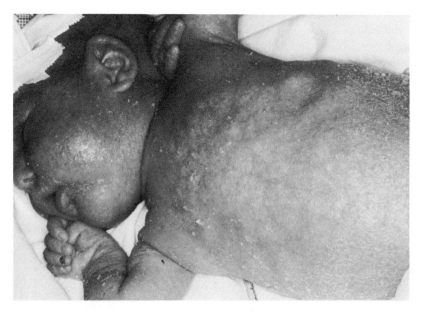

Figure 11 Severe exfoliant seborrheic dermatitis as seen in Leiner's disease. (*Source*: Ref. 2.)

eyebrows, and a thick profound exfoliation of the trunk and extremities. The scalp often if covered with thick, greasy, yellow crusts as seen in severe seborrheic dermatitis, and a patchy or total alopecia may be noted (Fig. 11). Although the course in some infants may be relatively benign, dehydration, fever, inanition, and death are not infrequent sequelae in patients with severe resistant forms of this disorder.

Infants with severe forms of familial Leiner's disease associated with generalized exfoliative dermatitis within 1 or 2 weeks of birth associated with severe diarrhea, recurrent gram-negative infections, wasting and death (similar to those originally described by Leiner) have been found to suffer from a defect in function of the fifth component of complement C_5. This dysfunction resulted in decreased phagocytosis (opsonic activity) of the patient's serum and resulted in failure to thrive and recurrent sepsis with an ominous prognosis. Whether or not infants with C_5 dysfunction syndrome represent true cases of Leiner's disease remains controversial [20].

DIAPER DERMATITIS

Diaper dermatitis is perhaps the most common cutaneous disorder of infancy and early childhood. Seen most frequently in infants and children less than 2 years of age, diaper dermatoses usually begin in the 1st and 2nd months of life and, if not properly controlled, may recur at intervals until the child no longer wears diapers.

The term "diaper rash" is used all too frequently in a diagnostic sense, as though the diverse dermatoses that may affect the anogenital region of infants

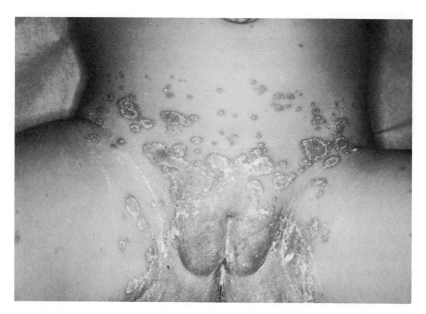

Figure 12 Candidal (monilial) diaper dermatitis. Beefy red erythema and satellite vesiculopustular lesions with white peripheral scale.

Table 7   Diaper Dermatitis

1. A symptom complex: a family of disorders
2. Etiology (a combination of factors):
   Prolonged contact or irritation to urine and feces
   Maceration due to wet diapers and impervious diaper coverings
   High incidence of secondary infection with *Candida albicans*

Source: Data from Ref. 2.

and young children constitute a single, specific clinical entity. Diaper dermatitis is not a specific diagnosis and is best viewed as a variable symptom complex, a family of disorders initiated by a combination of factors, the most significant being prolonged contact or irritation to the urine and feces, maceration engendered by wet diapers and impervious diaper coverings, and, in a high percentage of cases, secondary infection with underlying *Candida albicans* Table 7 and Fig. 12). Ammonia caused by bacterial breakdown of urea in the child's urine was thought to be a major factor in the etiology of diaper rash. Recent studies, however, refute the role of ammonia and urea-splitting bacteria in the etiology of this disorder [21,22].

GRANULOMA GLUTAEALE INFANTUM

Granuloma glutaeale infantum is a benign disorder of infancy characterized by reddish-purple granulomatous nodules which measure anywhere from 0.5 to 4.0 cm in diameter and occur in the groin, on the buttocks, lower aspect of the abdomen, penis, and intertriginous areas of the axillae and neck. Although the ominous appearance of these lesions may suggest a lymphomatous or sarcomatous process, the disorder appears to represent a unique cutaneous response to local inflammation, maceration, and secondary infection (usually *Candida albicans*) [23,24]. Since lesions of granuloma glutaeale infantum may resemble early lesions of Kaposi's sarcoma and may involve areas other than those of the diaper region, other names suggestive of this disorder include Kaposi's-sarcoma-like granuloma and granuloma intertriginosum infantum.

Granulomas may arise in a variety of infections; as allergic reactions to zirconium, in foreign body reactions; and in response to irritation, maceration, and infection in infants' intertriginous and diaper areas. Lesions of this disorder resolve completely and spontaneously within several months after treatment of the initiating inflammatory process with its associated maceration and secondary infection (Fig. 13).

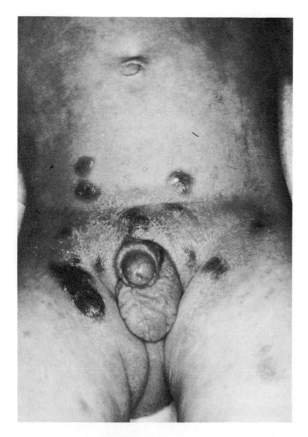

Figure 13 Granuloma glutaeale infantum. Ominous-appearing benign reddish-purple granulomatous nodules in the diaper area. (*Source*: Ref. 2.)

NEONATAL LUPUS ERYTHEMATOSUS

The lupus erythematosus (LE) cell factor can be transmitted via the placenta to infants born of mothers with lupus erythematosus. The maternal antibodies generally disappear and the LE test reverts to negative within the first 2 months of life. Congenital lupus also has been reported in children of unaffected as well as affected mothers with this disorder.

Infants born to mothers with disseminated LE are usually normal but have occasionally been found to have some manifestation of the disease, generally transient, including a discoid lupus rash, positive LE cell preparations, lymphocyte tuboreticular inclusions, and a syndrome of leukopenia, thrombocytopenia, and Coombs-test-positive hemolytic anemia.

It now appears that neonatal LE with discoid type lesions may not merely represent a transient disease and that systemic involvement and the development of congenital heart block or active and progressive lesions may be a distinct possibility in some infants with this disorder. These effects have been postulated to be due to immune complexes formed by transplacental passage of maternal antibodies. It is essential, therefore, that all children who have cutaneous neonatal LE be investigated for the possibility of congenital atrioventricular block and be followed for signs of active or recurring disease [25-27].

FUTURE CONSIDERATIONS

The diagnosis of heritable disease during early fetal life has made exciting progress in the past decade. Prenatal diagnosis has become a major adjunct to genetic counseling and is being used by thousands of couples to provide information by which they decide to either continue or terminate a pregnancy.

The most important technique for prenatal diagnosis has been amniocentesis to obtain amniotic fluid and the cells therein. These amniotic cells are fetal in origin and express considerable genetic information about the unborn child. Metabolic products from the fetus can be measured in the fluid, and chromosome examination and enzyme assays can be carried out with cultured amniotic cells. Homocystinuria, Fabry's disease, and the several mucopolysaccharidoses are examples of inborn areas of metabolism with skin manifestations that have been diagnosed prenatally. The challenge for the next decade is to broaden our comprehension of cutaneous pathophysiology and disease in infancy and early childhood, to "expand knowledge of human fetal development, to widen fetal diagnostic capabilities in early pregnancy, and to find ways to initiate treatment during fetal life" [28].

REFERENCES

1. Solomon LM, Esterly NB: Neonatal dermatology, in *Major Problems in Clinical Pediatrics, Volume IX*, edited by Schaffer AJ. Saunders, Philadelphia, 1973.
2. Hurwitz S: *Clinical Pediatric Dermatology. A Textbook of Skin Disorders of Childhood and Adolescence*. Saunders, Philadelphia, 1981.
3. Pillsbury DM: Pediatric dermatologic diagnosis, in *Dermatology*, edited by Moschella SL, Pillsbury DM, Hurley HJ Jr. Saunders, Philadelphia, 1975, pp 118-119.
4. Epstein WL: Contact-type delayed hypersensitivity in infants and children: induction of rhus sensitivity. Pediatrics 27:51-53, 1961.

5. Straus HW: Artificial sensitization of infants to poison ivy. J Allergy 2: 137-144, 1931.
6. Nachman RL, Esterly NB: Increased skin permeability in preterm infants. J Pediatr 79:628-632, 1971.
7. Committee on Fetus and Newborn: Skin care of the newly born infant, in *Standards and Recommendations for Hospital Care of Newborn Infants*, 6th Ed. American Academy of Pediatrics, Evanston, Illinois, 1977, pp 120-122.
8. Miller ME: *Host Defenses in the Human Neonate.* Grune & Stratton, New York, 1978.
9. South MA, Miller ME: Conversations on allergy and immunology. The inflammatory response in the newborn. Cutis 24:587-590, 1979.
10. Carr JA, Hodgman JD, Freeman RI, Levan NE: Relationship between toxic erythema and infant maturity. J Dis Child 112:129-134, 1966.
11. Eitzman DV, Smith RT: The non-specific inflammatory cycle in the neonatal infant. J Dis Child 97:326-334, 1959.
12. Ramamurthy RS, Riveri M, Esterly NB, Fretzin DF, Pildes RS: Transient neonatal pustular melanosis. J. Pediatr 88:831-835 (1976).
13. Torphy DE, Ray CG, McAlister R, Du JNH: Herpes simplex virus infection in infants: a spectrum of disease. J Pediatr 76:405-408, 1970.
14. Melish MC, Glasgow LA: Staphylococcal scalded skin syndrome: the expanded clinical syndrome. J Pediatr 78:958-967, 1971.
15. Wilkinson RH, Heller RM: Congenital syphilis: resurgence of an old problem. Pediatrics 47:27-30, 1971.
16. Warwick WJ, Ruttenberg HD, Quie PG: Sclerema neonatorum—a sign not a disease. JAMA 184:680-683, 1936.
17. Horsefield GI, Yardley HJ: Sclerema neonatorum. J Invest Dermatol 44: 326-336, 1965.
18. Marks MD: Subcutaneous adipose derangements of the newborn. Am J Dis Child 104:122-130, 1962.
19. Pochi PE, Strauss JS: Endocrinologic control of the development and activity of the human sebaceous gland. J Invest Dermatol 62:191-201, 1974.
20. Jacobs JC, Miller ME: Fatal familial Leiner's disease: a deficiency of the opsonic activity of serum complement. Pediatrics 49:225-232, 1972.
21. Leyden JJ, Katz S, Stewart R, Kligman AM: Urinary ammonia and ammonia-producing organisms in infants with and without diaper dermatitis. Arch Dermatol 113:1678-1680, 1977.
22. Leyden JJ, Kligman AM: The role of microorganisms in diaper dermatitis. Arch Dermatol 114:56-59, 1978.
23. Tappeiner J, Pfleger L: Granuloma glutaeale infantum. Hautarzt 22:383-388, 1971.
24. Uyeda K, Nakayasu K, Takaishi Y, Sotomatsu S: Kaposi Sarcoma-like granuloma—diaper dermatitis. A report of five cases. Arch Dermatol 107: 605-607, 1973.
25. Brustein D, Rodriguez JM, Minkin W, Rabhan NB: Familial lupus erythematosus. JAMA 238:2294-2296, 1977.

26. Chamiedes L, Truex RC, Vetter V, Rashkind WJ, Galioto FM, Jr, Noonan JA: Association of Maternal lupus erythematosus with congenital heart block. N Engl J Med 297:1204-1207, 1977.
27. Draznin TH, Esterly NB, Furey NL, DeBofsky H: Neonatal lupus erythematosus. J Am Acad Dermatol 1:437-442, 1979.
28. Research needs in 11 major areas of dermatology. Birth defects and genetic disorders. J Invest Dermatol 73:460-472, 1979.

Author Index

Subject Index